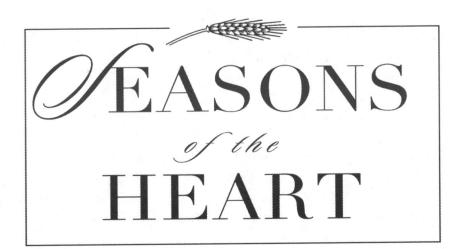

SEASONS *of the* HEART

Featuring the
Mediterranean-American Diet

With Foreword by Daniel E. Wise, MD, FACC

Presbyterian CARDIOVASCULAR INSTITUTE
CENTER FOR PREVENTIVE CARDIOLOGY

125 Baldwin Avenue, Suite 200
Charlotte, NC 28204
704-384-5043
www.presbyterian.org

To order additional copies, see order form in the back of this book or contact:

Presbyterian Center for Preventive Cardiology
125 Baldwin Avenue, Suite 200
Charlotte, NC 28204
704-384-5043
www.presbyterian.org

THE SEASON
OF OUR HEARTS...

For our patients and clients, it starts with a question: How can we improve our health?

For our staff, it begins with a passion to help others achieve their goals:
- Reduce their risk of cardiovascular disease
- Recover from a heart event
- Regain an optimal quality of life

The Center for Preventive Cardiology at Presbyterian Hospital's Cardiovascular Institute is dedicated to the mission of improving the health of our patients, clients, family and friends in our community. Programs and resources such as this cookbook are essential to enabling success. With education comes the knowledge that making lifestyle changes makes a difference in our health. Programs delivered with enthusiasm motivate people to set and take action toward their goals. Success

in achieving healthy lifestyle change builds excitement, renewed commitment and finally a total acceptance of a heart healthy lifestyle.

Our goals for everyone are to eat healthier, exercise daily and to balance priorities to minimize being overly stressed. We encourage everyone to embrace a healthier lifestyle!

Our first cookbook, *Eat Your Heart Out,* showed thousands of people that the Mediterranean-American Diet is delicious!

With great enthusiasm, we present *Seasons of the Heart*, our second cookbook designed for your enjoyment of the Mediterranean-American Diet. Featuring foods that are fresh each season, recipes range from very simple to elegant, yet all are easy to prepare. We're confident *Seasons of the Heart* will be another helpful resource for you and your family as you strive for a healthy heart and improved overall health.

Dedication

Seasons of the Heart is dedicated to our patients, clients and friends in our community and to the staff of our Center, as together, we embrace a heart healthier lifestyle.

Acknowledgments

Thank you to our core team who worked endless hours to make *Seasons of the Heart* a reality, Cheryl Kuhta-Sutter, RD, LDN, Mark Hoesten, RD, LDN and Nicole Martin.

Thank you to our Friends of the Heart, those patients, staff, family members and friends who donated favorite recipes for submission into our book. After analysis, some recipes were modified to meet dietary goals and all passed our taste tests. Your enthusiasm makes our cookbook special!

Jan Wagoner
Director

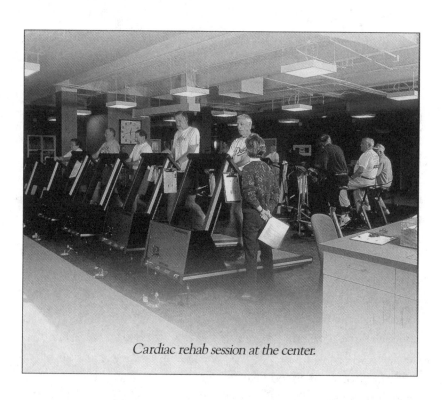

Cardiac rehab session at the center.

FOREWORD

The risk of cardiovascular disease is still the number one health problem in the United States and in the world. The risk of developing cardiovascular disease is in part driven by a genetic predisposition, but lifestyle plays a huge role in altering this predisposition in a positive way. Adopting a healthy lifestyle can markedly reduce the likelihood of having a heart attack, having a stroke, developing peripheral vascular disease or dying suddenly of a heart related problem. We have effective medications that help reduce risk, but research clearly indicates that the greatest benefit in reducing the risk of cardiovascular disease comes from adopting a healthy lifestyle that includes daily exercise and a healthy eating pattern.

The healthy eating pattern which has been best studied and produced the best results is the Mediterranean-American Diet. We have been teaching this diet for many years now and have seen outstanding results in patients who have adopted this program. The diet often leads to improvement in cardiovascular risk factors such as cholesterol, blood sugar and blood pressure. However, even in the absence of dramatic changes in these measures, the diet produces excellent overall health benefits and risk reduction. In the four large studies involving thousands of patients on the Mediterranean Diet, the most remarkable benefit of this diet was a decreased cardiovascular death rate from 44-76%.

The benefits of this diet are further enhanced by a consistent daily exercise program. We encourage everyone to try to exercise at least one hour each day. Ideally, this should be done in a single setting, but splitting the exercise into two or more sessions can be just as effective in reducing risk for cardiovascular disease. Studies have actually shown that using a pedometer and taking 10,000 steps per day has enormous medical benefits.

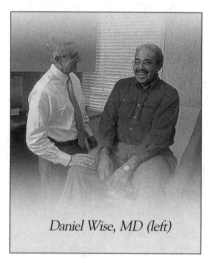

Daniel Wise, MD (left)

This new cookbook was created to augment our original cookbook, *Eat Your Heart Out.* The recipes are designed to use healthy seasonal produce to maximize the flavors each season offers us. The recipes all meet the dietary goals and the excellent tastes of the Mediterranean-American Diet! We hope you will find this cookbook as useful as our original cookbook and enjoy the recipes as much as we have enjoyed putting this together.

Daniel E. Wise, MD, FACC,
Diplomate, ABCL
Medical Director,
Presbyterian Center for
Preventive Cardiology

TABLE OF CONTENTS

Presbyterian) CARDIOVASCULAR INSTITUTE
CENTER FOR PREVENTIVE CARDIOLOGY

USING THE COOKBOOK

The Mediterranean Diet is based on the eating patterns of the people living in the lands of the Mediterranean Sea. The Mediterranean Diet has been studied for years. The people of the Mediterranean benefit from their healthy diets by having low rates of cardiovascular disease. The benefits are not from one specific food or nutrient; the benefits come from the combination of foods they eat. The Mediterranean Diet is rich in whole grains, fresh fruits and vegetables, fish and healthy fats.

Seasons of the Heart applies the dietary principals of the Mediterranean to the American diet. By combining the healthy aspects of a heart healthy American diet with the proven health benefits of the Mediterranean Diet, we can enjoy a better balance of nutrition and taste. The Mediterranean-American Diet is an eating plan, a lifestyle approach to food. Our patients and clients are proof that this way of living can be very delicious! Adopting the Mediterranean-American Diet allows us all to enjoy real food that tastes great and helps us to feel better every day. The added bonus is a healthier heart and improved overall health.

Enjoy the cookbook! Savor Stuffed Portabella Mushrooms on a brisk fall evening. Impress guests with a festive holiday Chocolate Éclair Cake. Enjoy a hot hearty bowl of Black Bean Chili on a cold winter day. Indulge with fresh Creamy Potato Salad on a warm spring afternoon. Relax with a cool refreshing Tomato Basil Salad on a hot summer day.

As decadent as these recipes sound, they are all designed and approved for individuals with heart disease and for those people who simply want to reduce their risk of heart disease and live a healthier lifestyle. Most recipes derive no more than 30% calories from fat, are very low in saturated fat and have little cholesterol. All goals of the Mediterranean-American Diet have been achieved. A few recipes may have a higher sodium content per serving than is recommended. However, with proper planning, these recipes can easily be enjoyed while maintaining a total recommended dietary sodium intake for the day. All recipes with a sodium content greater than 500 milligrams per serving are noted with a salt shaker in the heading of the recipe.

Choose from our selection of heart healthy recipes in *Seasons of the Heart.* These mouth watering recipes are arranged by the seasons, Winter, Spring, Summer and Autumn. A special Holiday section enables everyone to enjoy the season without compromising their Holiday traditions. All recipes are derived from delicious favorites and feature the freshest foods of the seasons. Within each section, recipes are arranged by appetizer, soup, salad, main dishes, vegetables, grains and desserts.

Enjoy these delicious recipes with confidence you are being true to your heart and improving your overall health.

Cookbook Symbols

Friends of the Heart

 Recipes displaying this symbol are favorite recipes donated by patients, staff, family members and friends. All recipes have been analyzed to meet dietary goals.

Sodium

 Recipes displaying this symbol are higher in sodium content and may need to be avoided by those on a sodium-restricted diet.

CHOOSE A HEALTHIER DIET

Diet is one of the most effective ways to decrease one's risk for cardiovascular disease and improve overall health. The fundamental dietary goals for reducing cardiovascular risk are:

- eat the right fats
- eat less cholesterol
- increase fiber and whole grains
- avoid excess sugar
- decrease sodium intake
- lose weight, if overweight

Eat the Right Fats

There are two types of fats: saturated and unsaturated. Saturated fat is one of the most harmful fats to the body because it stimulates LDL, or bad cholesterol, production. This type of fat is solid at room temperature and is found mostly in animal products such as beef, pork, poultry skin, high fat processed meats, whole milk products and butter. By choosing lean cuts of beef, trimming visible fat and choosing low fat dairy products, saturated fat can be reduced significantly.

Saturated fat is also found in a few vegetable oils including coconut, palm and palm kernel oil. Additional sources of this artery clogging fat are foods containing hydrogenated and partially hydrogenated oils. Hydrogenation is a process of transforming an unsaturated fat to a saturated fat, thus producing trans fatty acids. Hydrogenated oils are trans fats and should be avoided because they stimulate the production of bad blood fats. Specifically, they raise total cholesterol, raise LDL cholesterol and lower HDL cholesterol. If a product contains hydrogenated or partially hydrogenated oils, it will be located in the ingredient list. Since ingredients are listed in order by weight, choose products that have hydrogenated oils at the end of the list or none at all. A few foods that contain trans fats include margarine, breads, baked goods, snack foods and some cereals.

Unsaturated fats include 2 categories of fats, polyunsaturated and monounsaturated fats. These fats can decrease the risk of heart disease when they replace saturated fats. Unsaturated fats are liquid and don't raise cholesterol levels. Polyunsaturated fats lower LDL cholesterol in the blood. Unfortunately, polyunsaturated fats can also lower protective HDL cholesterol, thereby preventing some of the fat's beneficial effect. Polyunsaturated fats are found primarily in oils including safflower, sunflower, soybean, corn and sesame oils and also in some nuts and seeds.

One particular type of polyunsaturated fat called omega-3's decreases the risk for cardiovascular disease. Omega-3's reduce the stickiness of blood platelets, making them less likely to clump together and form harmful clots. Omega-3's also raise HDL cholesterol and lower triglycerides. Sources of omega-3 fatty acids include fatty fish such as salmon, mackerel, lake trout, cod and herring. Walnuts, canola oil and flaxseed are also rich in Omega-3's. To improve cardiac health, eat a minimum of three servings (15 ounces) of fish per week.

Monounsaturated fats are healthy because they reduce total cholesterol and LDL cholesterol while increasing HDL cholesterol. Sources of monounsaturated fats include olive and canola oils, avocados and almonds. Choose these fats whenever possible.

Eat Less Cholesterol

Cholesterol is necessary for life. The body uses cholesterol to build strong membranes, steroids, estrogen, testosterone and to ensure adequate function of the nervous system. The body makes all the cholesterol it needs to function. Therefore, dietary cholesterol is not necessary. On the contrary, excess blood cholesterol and other blood fats are harmful because they lead to the formation of fatty plaques. Fatty plaques can lead to narrowing of the arteries, "blockages" and clots. When dietary cholesterol and saturated fat are limited, blood cholesterol levels are reduced. Cholesterol is only found in animal products: meat, fish, poultry and dairy products. Dietary cholesterol can be reduced by choosing lean cuts of beef such as filet mignon, eye of round and London broil. When buying chicken or turkey, choose skinless white meat only. Be aware of labels claiming "no cholesterol." Products that don't contain cholesterol may contain other types of harmful fats such as partially hydrogenated oils. Remember, cholesterol is found ONLY in animal products. Trans fats and other saturated fats have a greater negative impact on cardiovascular health than dietary cholesterol.

Eat More Fiber

There are two types of fiber, soluble and insoluble. Soluble fiber aids in cholesterol reduction and blood sugar control whereas insoluble fiber provides roughage to help the digestive track run smoothly. Because it creates a feeling of being full, fiber helps to control weight. It also passes through the digestive tract faster and as a result, the body absorbs fewer calories. Since the average American diet lacks adequate fruit, vegetables and whole grains, it falls short of the 25-35 grams of fiber recommended per day. To boost dietary fiber, choose whole grains over refined grains. Whole grains contain all parts of the fiber kernel: the bran, germ and endosperm. Refined grains lack most of the bran and germ. Therefore, refined grains have little or no fiber. Examples of whole grains to include in one's diet are whole wheat pasta, brown rice, whole grain cereals, whole oats, whole wheat crackers and whole wheat breads. When choosing starches, be sure the first word in the ingredient list is WHOLE and not unbleached, enriched, wheat or white flour.

Eat Less Sugar

Excess sugar in the diet can lead to weight gain, elevated triglycerides, decreased HDL cholesterol and uncontrolled blood sugar levels. The average American consumes more than 25% of daily calories from sugar. Only one-third of this sugar is from sucrose or table sugar while the rest comes from processed foods and beverages. Sugar is found not only in table sugar, but also in fruit juice, fruit, honey, molasses, desserts (especially fat free desserts), soda, alcohol, cereal, white potatoes, white rice, white pasta and other starches made from white flour. Sugar is described by many names such as brown sugar, cane sugar, corn syrup, high fructose corn syrup, honey, lactose, maple syrup and sugar alcohols (mannitol, sorbitol and xylitol). Some of the most common sources of sugar to **LIMIT OR AVOID** in the diet include:

- Table sugar, brown sugar and powdered sugar
- All types of candy and gum
- Cakes, cookies and pies including fat-free desserts
- Commercially baked breads, pastries, crackers and rolls
- Processed foods such as tomato sauce, spaghetti sauce and baked beans
- Many breakfast cereals, especially those containing fruit
- Refined grains such as white rice, white potatoes and white pasta
- Yogurt
- Canned fruits
- Jams and jellies
- Salad dressings, marinades and ketchup
- Sweetened tea, fruit juice, soda, punch, fruit cocktail beverages and chocolate milk
- Alcohol

Aim for 7 grams of "sugars" per serving on food labels and limit total consumption of "sugars" to 40 or less grams per day. The Food and Drug Administration has approved several artificial sweeteners to replace sugar in many foods and beverages thereby decreasing total calories.

Eat Less Sodium

Excess sodium in the diet

elevates blood pressure and increases our risk of stroke and other cardiovascular disease. Patients with known congestive heart failure should be very careful to limit sodium intake because fluid balance is very important to maintaining a stable heart. Although national guidelines suggest 2300 milligrams or less of sodium per day, individuals with cardiovascular disease or at risk for cardiovascular disease should eat 2000 milligrams or less of sodium each day, which is equal to about one teaspoon of salt.

Lose Weight, If Overweight

Carrying too much weight increases risk for heart and other cardiovascular diseases, diabetes, hypertension, stroke, gallbladder and other diseases. Apple shaped individuals are those who tend to carry their excess body weight in the abdomen. This belly fat increases their risk for cardiovascular disease, diabetes and other health risks. Sixty percent of American adults are overweight or obese. More and more Americans are turning to fast food restaurants, processed foods and fat free snacks and desserts due to hectic schedules and lack of meal planning. Consequently, the United States is seeing a steady increase in childhood obesity, diabetes and cardiovascular disease. To reduce health risks, we must adopt a healthier diet and exercise regularly.

MEDITERRANEAN FOOD GUIDE PYRAMID

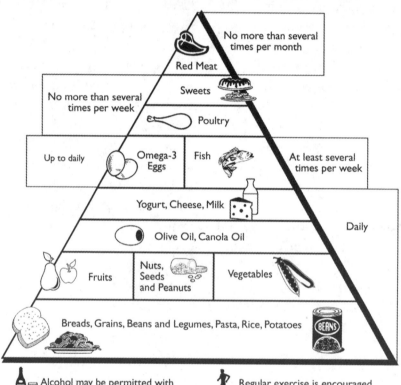

Red Meat — No more than several times per month

Sweets

Poultry — No more than several times per week

Omega-3 Eggs — Up to daily

Fish — At least several times per week

Yogurt, Cheese, Milk

Olive Oil, Canola Oil

Daily

Fruits

Nuts, Seeds and Peanuts

Vegetables

Breads, Grains, Beans and Legumes, Pasta, Rice, Potatoes

Alcohol may be permitted with meals as approved by your physician

Regular exercise is encouraged as approved by your physician

UNDERSTANDING FATS

Healthy Lifestyles

As you adopt a heart healthy diet, please remember these are lifestyle changes. This nutrition plan is not a short-term diet, but should be maintained for life.

As you begin your journey to become healthier, we encourage you to become aware of food labels. Please take a minute while you are grocery shopping to read food labels and pay special attention to the ingredients list.

Know Your Fats

By decreasing the amount of saturated fat and avoiding trans fat in your diet, your risk of cardiovascular disease, cancer, diabetes, high cholesterol levels, hypertension and obesity will be reduced. Learning about the types of fats can help you make healthier low-fat food choices:

- **Cholesterol** – Cholesterol is found only in animal products (meat and dairy products).
- **Unsaturated fat** – Fat that

is liquid at room temperature; primarily plant sources. Unsaturated fat is a better choice than saturated fat.

Polyunsaturated fat – Helps to lower total cholesterol and LDL; it contains essential fatty acids (EFA), which the body doesn't make. Examples include corn, soybean, sunflower, vegetable and soybean oils, Omega-3 fatty acids, walnuts, flax and fish.

Monounsaturated fat – Helps to lower total cholesterol and LDL; this may also help to raise HDL levels. Examples include canola oil, olive oil and peanut oils, almonds and nuts.

- **Saturated fat** – Fat that is solid at room temperature; mostly found in animal products. Examples include lard, butter, chocolate, palm kernel and coconut oils, marbled red meat, dark meat (from chicken and turkey), whole and 2% milk, full fat cheese, cream and fried foods. Note: Palm kernel and coconut oils are highly saturated even though they are of vegetable origin.

- **Hydrogenated** – Plastic at room temperature. Hydrogenation is a process that makes an unsaturated fat more saturated. As a result of hydrogenation, trans fatty acids are produced. Trans fats are a harmful fat that should be eliminated from the diet. Trans fatty acids are included in the total fat content on food labels. When reading a food label, trans fats should always read zero. Hydrogenated or partially hydrogenated fats are found in fried foods, crackers, pastries, cakes, cookies, snack foods, some breads and cereals and prepackaged food items. Look at the ingredient list to find hydrogenated or partially hydrogenated oils. If either are listed, please make sure it is located at the end of the ingredient list.

Improving Lipid Levels with Good Nutrition

Dietary suggestions that can help improve lipids and overall health:

- **Watch portion sizes!** An appropriate serving of any type of meat is three ounces (size of a deck of cards). You can follow a low fat diet and gain weight or increase lipid concentrations by overeating the good stuff too, such as too many carbohydrates, too much fruit, etc.
- **Limit red meat** (beef, veal, lamb and pork) to six ounces a week, or less.
- **Aim for 15 oz of fish** (tuna, trout, salmon, mackerel, halibut, cod, anchovy, swordfish, sardines or white fish) per week.
- **Increase your intake of legumes** (peas and beans). These are very low in fat and contain a large amount of fiber.
- **Eat the majority of your foods during the day** when you are more active and less in the evening when your activity level is lower.
- **Eat several meals or snacks throughout the day,** instead of a few large meals.
- **Choose more whole grain products and limit refined grains.** When reading a food label, please refer to the

ingredient list. Make sure the very first word is whole. If the first word is not whole (for example, the first word is enriched or unbleached), the product is not whole grain and should be limited in the diet. Whole grains have much more fiber, whereas refined grains have been processed and are missing most of the fiber from the whole-wheat kernel. Refined grains lack nutrients and have a tendency to raise blood sugar and triglycerides due to their sugar content.

Examples of whole grains include: whole-wheat pasta, brown rice, Shredded Wheat®, Bran Flakes®, Total®, Cheerios®, All-Bran®, oatmeal, brown rice, whole wheat breads and oats

Examples of refined grains include: white flour products (white pasta, white rice), Special K®, Cornflakes®, grits, Cream of Wheat®, Rice Krispies®, white breads and many types of crackers (Saltines®, Townhouse®, etc.)

DIETARY RECOMMENDATIONS TO LOWER TRIGLYCERIDES AND BLOOD SUGAR

Goals

- Avoid simple sugars especially in sweetened beverages and desserts. Replace white flour starches with whole wheat and whole grains.
- Choose whole fruit instead of juice and limit fruit to 3 servings per day.
- Avoid alcohol.
- Choose foods with 7 grams or less of "sugars" per serving and less than 40 grams of "sugars" per day.

Meats and Fish

CHOOSE: White meat chicken and turkey breast; fresh or frozen fish (unbreaded) and fish canned in water; lean red meat with any excess fat trimmed (eye of round, London broil, flank steak, filet mignon, Canadian bacon, 96% or leaner ground beef).
AVOID: Skin, fat and dark meat of chicken and turkey; organ meats; marbled beef (such as ribeye, porterhouse); processed meats (such as hotdogs, sausage, bologna); fatty fowl.

Dairy and Eggs

CHOOSE: Soy, skim, 1/2 or 1% milk; "light" refrigerated yogurt without fruit and less than 11 grams of "sugars"; low fat and fat free cheeses; egg substitutes and egg whites (use freely); omega-3 eggs (1 yolk per day).
AVOID: 2% and whole milk; whole milk puddings, yogurt or cheeses; non-dairy substitutes; more than two regular egg yolks per week.

Nuts and Beans

CHOOSE: Two tablespoons or less per day of natural peanut butter, trans fat free peanut butter, 1 ounce of nuts (preferably walnuts, almonds or peanuts); dried, canned or frozen peas or beans (black-eyed peas, navy beans, kidney, pinto, soy and black beans).

LIMIT: Processed peanut butter, cashews; lima beans and commercial baked beans.

Fruits

CHOOSE: Two to three servings per day of fresh fruit or canned fruit packed in water, in its own juice or EXTRA light syrup.

LIMIT: Frozen fruit and fruit canned in light/heavy syrup; bananas, watermelon, pineapple, coconut, raisins and other dried fruits. Avoid ALL fruit juice.

Vegetables

CHOOSE: All vegetables, especially those with dark and vibrant colors.

LIMIT: Starchy vegetables which include: white potatoes (in all forms), corn (and corn products), lima beans, carrots and green peas.

Breads and Grains

CHOOSE: Whole wheat and whole grain breads and cereals (such as Shredded Wheat®, oatmeal, Bran Flakes®, Cheerios®, Wheat Chex®, Wheaties®, GrapeNuts®); whole wheat pasta; brown rice; bulgar,

bran and wheat germ. The first word in the product's ingredient list needs to read **whole.**

AVOID: Any bread that is not made from 100% whole wheat flour (cornbread, hamburger buns, French bread, etc.); all sweetened cereals; white pasta and white rice; white flour.

Desserts and Snacks

CHOOSE OFTEN: Whole grain crackers (Triscuits®, Wasa®, Ry Krisp®, Finn Crisp®, Ryvita®, Wheatettes®, Ak-Mak®), popcorn (air popped or stove top), whole grain cereal, nuts, no sugar added fruitbars/fudgesicles; sugar free puddings made with skim milk; sugar free Jello®.

LIMIT: Pretzels, whole grain snacks with hydrogenated fat (microwave popcorn), animal crackers, graham crackers, light AND no sugar added ice cream.

AVOID: Fried snack foods (potato chips); "white flour" crackers with hydrogenated fat (Saltines®, Ritz® and many more); regular, light and fat free ice cream or frozen yogurt, sherbet, sorbet; whole milk puddings; ALL cookies, cakes, pies, pastries and other "dessert" type foods.

Fats, Oils and Condiments

CHOOSE: Margarine or butter that is fat free or "trans fat free", Benecol Light®, Smart Balance® or Take Control® margarine; olive and canola oils; low fat or fat free mayonnaise; fat-free, light or vinaigrette salad dressings; light or sugar free syrup and no sugar added jellies/jams.

AVOID: Saturated fat found in butter, lard, animal fats, bacon drippings, gravies, cream sauces; palm kernel and coconut oils; regular mayonnaise and salad dressings; regular syrup, jellies and jams.

Beverages

CHOOSE: Water; coffee; plain or herbal teas; diet soda; "sugar free" drinks.

AVOID: Fruit juice and juice cocktails; regular soda; sweetened tea and drinks (Kool-Aid®); sports drinks (Gatorade®); alcohol.

STUDY THE LABEL – IT CAN HELP YOU CHOOSE THE RIGHT FOODS

Sample Ingredient List

An ingredient list is simply a list of what a food item contains. They are listed in order by weight. Every food label is required to have one; here is a sample:

What if there are two or more fats listed on the label?

Products may have more than one fat in the ingredient list. They are listed in order by weight. The first fat listed is in the largest amount. It is best to avoid any product that contains a fat listed on the "to avoid" list.

Does the kind of fat always matter?

Yes! Healthy fats include mono and poly unsaturated fats. Unhealthy fats are saturated and trans fats. Trans fats will be indicated by the words "hydrogenated oil" and "partially hydrogenated oil" in the ingredient list. Packages that say "No trans fat per serving" may still contain hydrogenated oil. Products that contain NO hydrogenated oil are preferred. However, if products contain hydrogenated oil, they should be at the end of the ingredient list.

Nutrition Facts

Serving Size 1 cup (55g)
Servings Per Container 5

Amount Per Serving	Cereal	Cereal with 1/2 cup Skim Milk
Calories	190	230
Calories from Fat	40	40
		% Daily Value
Total Fat 5g	8%	3%
Saturated Fat 0.5g	3%	3%
Trans Fat 0g		
Cholesterol 0mg	0%	0%
Sodium 135mg	6%	8%
Total Carbohydrate 38g	13%	15%
Dietary Fiber 10g	40%	40%
Sugars less than 1g		
Protein 7g		

Uncle Sam Cereal®

Ingredients: Whole Wheat Kernels, Whole Flaxseed, Salt, Barley Malt, Niacin, Riboflavin (Vitamin B2), Thiamin Mononitrate (Vitamin B2).

What fats should you look for?

Use Mostly	Avoid
• Olive oil	• Butter
• Canola oil	• Lard
• Peanut oil	• Bacon or Bacon fat
	• Vegetable Shortening
Use Sparingly	• Coconut oil
• Safflower oil	• Palm kernel oil
• Sunflower oil	• Cottonseed oil
	• Trans fat (hydrogenated oil)

More Helpful Hints

- Limit the total fat to 3 grams for every 100 calories
- Limit saturated fat to 12 grams or less per day or 1/4 of total fat per serving
- Ignore cholesterol
- Limit sodium to 2300 mg per day; 2000 mg for those with hypertension or with a history of congestive heart failure
- Aim for 25-35 grams of fiber per day; choose products with 3 or more grams of fiber per serving
- Limit "sugars" to 7 grams or less per serving; total "sugars" to 40 grams or less per day

LABEL CLAIMS –
WHAT DO THEY REALLY MEAN?

FDA Regulations

Label claims are regulated by the FDA and must meet certain criteria for use. Claims can be inadvertently misleading because they tend not to tell the whole story. You may still need to check the ingredients or look at other nutrients on the Nutrition Facts label before you choose the product. The following chart is provided from the FDA website, www.fda.gov.

Label Claim Definitions

Label Claim	Definition	Be Aware
Fat-free	Less than 0.5 grams of fat per serving	Check the ingredient list to be sure that the fat is the recommended type. If not, choose a product with less than one gram of total fat on the Nutrition Facts label. The product may still be high in sugar.
Low-fat	3 grams of total fat or less per serving	
Reduced fat	At least 25% less fat per serving than reference food	
Saturated fat-free	Less than 0.5 grams of saturated fat and less than 0.5 grams of trans fatty acids per serving	
Low saturated fat	1 gram of saturated fat or less per serving	
Reduced saturated fat	At least 25% less than reference food and 2 grams or less of saturated fat per serving	
Cholesterol-free	Less than 2 mg cholesterol and 2 grams or less saturated fat per serving	
Low-cholesterol	20 mg cholesterol or less and 2 grams or less saturated fat per serving	
Reduced cholesterol	At least 25% less cholesterol than reference food and 2 grams or less saturated fat per serving	
No Trans Fatty Acids or Trans fat-free	Product must contain less than 0.5 grams per serving of trans fatty acids	
Lean	Less than 10 grams of total fat and 4.5 grams or less of saturated fat	Used for labeling of meat, poultry, seafood or game. Products labeled "Extra Lean" are usually acceptable.
Extra Lean	Less than 5 grams of fat and less than 2 grams of saturated fat	
High Fiber	5 grams or more of fiber per serving	Foods with a fiber claim must also be "low fat" or the total fat per serving must appear next to the claim.
Good source of fiber	2.5 to 4.9 grams of fiber per serving	
More or added fiber	At least 2.5 grams more fiber per serving than the reference food	
Whole Wheat	A grain milled in its entirety (all but the husk), not refined.	The first grain ingredient should be whole wheat, whole grain or whole oat.

RECIPE SUBSTITUTIONS

Instead of...	Try...
Whole or 2% milk	Skim, 1/2% or 1% milk or soy milk
Heavy cream	Evaporated skim milk
Whipped cream	Nonfat whipped topping
Cream cheese	Fat free cream cheese
Sour cream	Nonfat or low fat sour cream or plain nonfat yogurt
Cheese	Part skim cheese made with 2% milk or soy cheese
Whole egg	Two egg whites
Baking chocolate (1 oz square)	3 tablespoons cocoa powder plus one tablespoon canola oil
Fudge sauce	Light chocolate syrup
Regular margarine	Trans fat free margarine
Shortening or butter	Trans fat free margarine; olive or canola oil
Vegetable oil	Olive or canola oil
Oil in baked goods	Equal amounts of unsweetened applesauce
Mayonnaise	Mustard, low fat mayonnaise or fat free mayonnaise
Gravy	Gravy made with bouillon cubes; low fat broth thickened with flour or cornstarch; commercial fat free gravy
Cream soup	Low fat or fat free, reduced sodium varieties
Real bacon bits/bacon	Imitation bacon bits; turkey bacon or Canadian bacon
Salt	Reduce the amount by half; try light salt or salt substitutes
Oil packed tuna	Water packed tuna
Regular ground beef	96% lean ground beef
Ground turkey	Ground turkey breast or 99% lean ground turkey

FIBER

There are two types of fiber:

- **Insoluble** – Provides roughage to help the digestive system run smoothly (bran, whole grains, cabbage, broccoli, apples, carrots, etc.)
- **Soluble** – Helps to decrease cholesterol and control glucose levels (oats, squash, apples, citrus fruits, berries, breakfast cereals, etc.)

Good Sources of Fiber

Dietary recommendation – 25-35 grams per day

Food + Serving Size	Fiber Grams	Fat Grams	Food + Serving Size	Fiber Grams	Fat Grams
Blackberries, 1/2 cup	5.3	1	Black-eyed peas, 1/2 cup	10	
Raisins, 1/4 cup	4.5		Pinto beans, 1/2 cup	10	
Pear with skin, 1 med	4.3	1	Kidney beans, 1/2 cup	9.5	
Strawberries, 1 cup	4	1	Navy beans, 1/2 cup	8	
Blueberries, 1 cup	4	1	Lima beans, 1/2 cup	8	
Raspberries, 1/2 cup	4		Black beans, 1/2 cup	6.5	
Kiwi, 1	3		Baked beans, 1/2 cup	6	1
Orange, 1 medium	3		Great northern, 1/2 cup	5.5	2
Apple w/ skin, 1 med	3		Chick peas, 1/2 cup	5	
Apricots, 3 medium	2.3	1	Lentils, 1/2 cup	5	
Peaches, 1 medium	2.1		Green peas, 1/2 cup	4.2	
Grapefruit, one-half	2		All Bran Xtra Fiber®, 1/2 cup	14	1
Banana, 1 medium	2	1	Fiber One®, 1/2 cup	13	
Grapefruit, one-half	2		All Bran®, 1/3 cup	10	
Broccoli, cooked, 1 cup	6	1	Fiber 1 Honey Clusters®	14	
Brussel sprouts, 1cup	6		Post Raisin Bran®, 2/3 cup	6	1
Potato with skin, 1 med	5	1	Total Raisin Bran®, 1 cup	6	
Cabbage, 1 cup cooked	4		Shredded Wheat®, 1 cup	5	
Zucchini, 1 cup cooked	4		MultiGrain Cheerios®, 1 cup	3	1
Sweet potato, 1 med	3.5	1	Grape Nuts®, 1/4 cup	2	
Carrots, cooked, 1/2 cup	3		100% whole wheat bread, 1 slice	3	1
Spinach, cooked, 1/2 cup	2.5		Popcorn, 3 cups	3	Varies
Corn, 1/2 cup	3	1	Whole wheat pasta, 1/2 cup	6	1
Tomato, raw, 1 med	2				
Brown rice, 1/2 cup	3	2			

Whole Grain vs. Refined Grain

- **Whole grain** – contains the bran (which is comprised of selenium, copper and other antioxidants), fiber, vitamins and minerals.

A product is a whole grain if the label or ingredient says: whole wheat or whole grain.

- **Refined grain** – most of the bran and germ have been removed through processing (usually leaves very little fiber). A product is a refined grain if the label or ingredient list says: cracked wheat, multi-grain, oat bran, seven-bran, made with whole wheat, made with whole grain, rye (breads), stoned wheat, wheat and whole bran.

Examples of Whole and Refined Grains

- **Whole grains** – Cheerios®, Mueslix®, Grape Nuts®, Shredded Wheat®, Total®, Wheat Germ®, Wheaties®, All Bran®, Bran Flakes®, oatmeal, whole-wheat pasta and brown rice.
- **Refined grains** – Basic 4®, Cornflakes®, Rice Krispies®, Frosted Flakes®, Product 19®, Puffed Wheat®, Special K®, Cream of Wheat®, grits, white rice, white pasta, Saltines® and other "white flour" products.

When increasing fiber intake, do so gradually and drink plenty of water.

Choose more whole grains for satiety, less sugar and to help lower total cholesterol.

SODIUM

The average American consumes 4000-6000 milligrams of sodium each day. Too much sodium in the diet elevates blood pressure and increases our risk for stroke and other cardiovascular diseases. In individuals with a history of congestive heart failure or hypertension, limit sodium intake to less than 2000 milligrams daily. For others, sodium intake of 2300 milligrams a day is recommended.

There are many sodium rich foods which are obvious to the consumer but there are also a good number of products with hidden sodium that need to be avoided as well. These include:

- Condiments such as ketchup, soy sauce, bouillon cubes, salad dressings and marinades
- Herbs and spices that contain salt, such as garlic salt
- Salt as a garnish in alcoholic drinks
- Processed luncheon meats
- Most canned and frozen foods
- Cheese
- Tomato juice and other breakfast drinks
- Spaghetti and tomato sauces
- Fast food, such as french fries and hamburgers
- Snack foods and many desserts
- Butter and margarine
- Cereals, breads, frozen pancakes and waffles
- Antacids

Aim for 2000-2300 milligrams or less of sodium each day which is almost the equivalent of one teaspoon of salt. When reading food labels, use the following sodium guidelines:

- Low sodium is 140 milligrams or less per serving
- Very low sodium is 35 milligrams or less per serving
- Sodium free is 5 milligrams or less per serving

POTASSIUM

Potassium plays a major role in maintaining fluid and electrolyte balance, nerve transmissions and muscle contractions within the body's cells. A normal serum potassium level is 3.5 to 5.5 mEq/L. The recommended intake of potassium for adults is approximately 2000 mg/day. The following is a list of potassium rich foods:

Potassium-Rich Foods

Food	Serving Size	Potassium (mg)
Figs, dried	10	1331
Soybeans, roasted and salted	1/2 cup	1173
Chili with beans, canned	1 cup	931
Pumpkin seeds, roasted and salted	1/2 cup	915
Baked potato with skin	1	825
100% Bran cereal	1 cup	652
Halibut, baked	4 oz	636
Pistachio's dry roasted, salted, shelled	1/2 cup	620
Baked potato without skin	1	610
Snapper, baked/broiled	4 oz	590
Yogurt, made with skim milk	1 cup	579
Grouper, baked	4 oz	537
Tomato juice	1 cup	537
Plain yogurt	1 cup	531
Bass, baked/broiled	4 oz	515
Cod, poached	4 oz	496
Lima beans, cooked	1/2 cup	478
Winter squash, baked	1/2 cup	448
Salmon, baked/broiled	4 oz	425
Artichoke	1	425
Cantaloupe	1/4 melon	412
Milk, low fat	1 cup	400
Pinto beans, cooked	1/2 cup	400
Banana	1	400
Sweet potato, baked in skin	1	397
Soybeans, cooked	1/2 cup	390

Potassium-Rich Foods, continued

Food	Serving Size	Potassium (mg)
Broccoli, cooked	1/2 cup	374
Post Raisin Bran®	1 cup	355
Almonds, dry roasted	1/3 cup	354
Prune juice	1/2 cup	351
Honeydew	1/10 melon	350
Tomatoes, cooked	1/2 cup	346
Turkey, white meat	4 oz	346
Avocado	1/4 cup	344
Soymilk	1 cup	338
Peanuts, oil roasted	1/3 cup	335
Navy beans, cooked	1/2 cup	335
Grape juice	1 cup	334
Kidney beans, cooked	1/2 cup	330
Blackeyed peas	1/2 cup	319
Nectarine	1 medium	300
Tomato	1 fresh	300
All Bran Cereal®	1/3 cup	284
Spinach, frozen, cooked	1/2 cup	283
Potatoes, mashed	1/2 cup	274
Orange	1 medium	265
Kiwi	1	252
Orange juice	1/2 cup	248
Garbanzo beans, cooked	1/2 cup	235
Prunes	5 medium	224
Apricots, canned in juice	1/2 cup	205

ARE YOU AT RISK FOR CARDIOVASCULAR DISEASE?

Do you know your risk of cardiovascular disease; that is, your risk of having a heart attack, stroke, or need for a cardiac procedure, such as a heart cath, angioplasty or coronary artery bypass surgery? Did you know that pain in your legs while walking can be due to vascular disease, the same disease process that causes heart attacks?

Take the survey below. Check any statement that is true for you. Talk with your physician about your personal risk.

Risk Factors

A risk factor is a factor or element that can cause damage or disease.

Non-Modifiable Risk Factors

Risk factors that cannot be changed:

- **Gender** – Men are at greater risk for cardiovascular disease than women until women reach menopause. Then a woman's risk is the same as that of a man.
- **Age** – The risk of cardiovascular disease increases as a person ages. Males older than 45 years and females older than 55 years are at increased risk.
- **Genetics** – Family history of premature heart disease increases risk.

Modifiable Risk Factors

Factors that can be changed and modified:

- **Tobacco/Smoking** – Tobacco use/smoking is the number one modifiable risk factor. Nicotine present in tobacco products is a stimulant and constrictor, which increases blood pressure, heart rate and clotting tendencies. Tobacco use stresses the heart muscle.
- **Abnormal Lipid Values** – High LDL, high LDL particle concentration, low HDL,

elevated triglycerides, elevated total cholesterol, elevated Lp(a) and elevated homocysteine levels increase a person's risk for cardiovascular disease. Ideal values:

Total cholesterol < 160 mg/d
LDL < 70 mg/dl
HDL > 60 mg/dl (men),
    > 65 mg/dl (women)
Triglycerides < 80 mg/dl

- **Diabetes** – Diabetes ages the body and arteries at an accelerated rate.

- **Hypertension** – Blood pressure (BP) of greater than 135/85 mm/Hg, a condition referred to as hypertension, is considered too high. Elevated BP overworks the heart and can lead to heart and kidney failure. Ideal BP: <120/<80mmhg

- **Sedentary Lifestyle** – Results in elevated blood fat/lipid levels, low energy and elevated resting and exercise heart rates, which indicate an inefficient heart muscle.

- **High Fat, Low Nutrition Diet** – Leads to elevated weight and lipid levels.

- **Obesity** – Elevated body weight increases the workload on the heart.

- **Metabolic Syndrome** – a condition that is diagnosed by any 3 of the 5 risk factors including hypertension, elevated triglycerides, low HDL cholesterol and being overweight as defined by either abdominal circumference greater than 35 inches for women and 40 inches for men or a body mass index (BMI) greater than 24.9.

- **Stress** – Stress can be a significant factor in the development of cardiovascular disease. Chronic stress stimulates the release of stress hormones which lead to increased heart rate, constriction of arteries, elevated blood pressure and an increase in the clotting of the blood.

EXERCISE FOR LIFE

Consistent exercise is an important part of achieving a heart healthy lifestyle. Together, with healthy eating and stress management, your risk factors can be reduced and your overall health improved. The benefits of exercise include:

- Stronger heart
- Increased energy
- Weight loss/weight maintenance
- Better control of diabetes, blood pressure and blood lipids
- Feeling better and more relaxed

Before beginning your exercise program, ask your physician for medical clearance. It is important to find an activity that you enjoy. You don't have to join a gym to exercise. Walking is one of the easiest, most cost effective types of aerobic activity. You can walk anywhere, on a treadmill, around your neighborhood or in a mall. Use a pedometer to count your steps; your goal is 10,000 steps per day. An excellent long term goal would be to walk about 20 miles per week.

Please treat exercise like medicine. For best results, exercise daily. Gradually increase your exercise time daily until you can exercise at least 60 minutes every day.

Your exercise session should include the following:

- **Warm-up** – begin each exercise session with an 8-10 minute warm-up. Example: if you are walking, walk slowly for 8-10 minutes. If you are cycling, cycle slowly for 8-10 minutes.
- **Aerobic activity** – 20-60 minutes of moderate activity. Aerobic exercise means moving large muscle groups continuously. Some examples of aerobic activities include: walking, jogging, cycling, dancing and swimming.

- **Cool down** – your cool down should last 8-10 minutes and can be as simple as the warm-up: gradually slow the pace and intensity of your chosen activity.
- **Stretching** – stretch at the end of your exercise session while your muscles are warm and more pliable. Try to hold each stretch for 15-60 seconds.

Consistent efforts are the keys to success in making healthy lifestyle changes. Here are some quick tips to get you on your way to an active and safe lifestyle:

- Drink 8 ounces of water before, during (every 20 minutes) and at least 16 ounces after activities.
- Exercise indoors if the weather is too hot; that is, if the sum of humidity plus the temperature (Fahrenheit degrees) is greater than 150.
- Exercise indoors if the weather is too cold; that is, if the temperature is less than 40° actual or with wind chill.
- Do not exercise immediately following a meal. Allow two hours for sufficient digestion.
- Exercise should not be painful; work at a level that you feel is *light* to *somewhat* hard.

In conclusion, exercise is one of the most important medicinal therapies known to man! Embrace these guidelines to develop or enhance a safe exercise program.

Please use this cookbook to serve delicious, easy to prepare recipes as well as a guide to improve your overall health!

STRESS

Stress is a complex, dynamic process of interaction between a person and his or her life. It is the way we react physically, mentally and emotionally to the various conditions, changes and demands of life. We know that certain amounts of stress are motivational. However, problems begin to occur when we do not deal with our stress in a healthy fashion.

The following are some of the symptoms that you may experience when under stress:

- Low energy level
- Overeating/under eating
- Gritting teeth
- Queasy stomach, nausea, vomiting
- Muscles aches
- Insomnia
- Rapid heartbeat
- Irritability
- Smoking

It is very important to adopt healthy coping techniques to deal with stress. Something as simple as breathing is an excellent way to relieve stress in your everyday life. Whether you are sitting in your office or stuck in traffic, you can focus your attention on your breath and practice breathing techniques. Simply inhaling for a count of 2 and exhaling for a count of 4 is a fantastic way to relieve stress.

The following are several other healthy coping techniques that you may want to try:

- Massage therapy
- Progressive muscle relaxation
- Regular exercise
- Maintain a well balanced diet (Mediterranean-American Diet) low in fat, sugar and salt with adequate fiber
- Talk about your feelings to someone you trust
- Accept your limitations
- Ask for and accept help
- Learn how to say "NO"
- Laugh and cry
- Rest and relax
- Look for the beauty and blessings in life

Whatever technique you enjoy, use it. Practicing healthy coping techniques is an essential part of achieving optimal heart health.

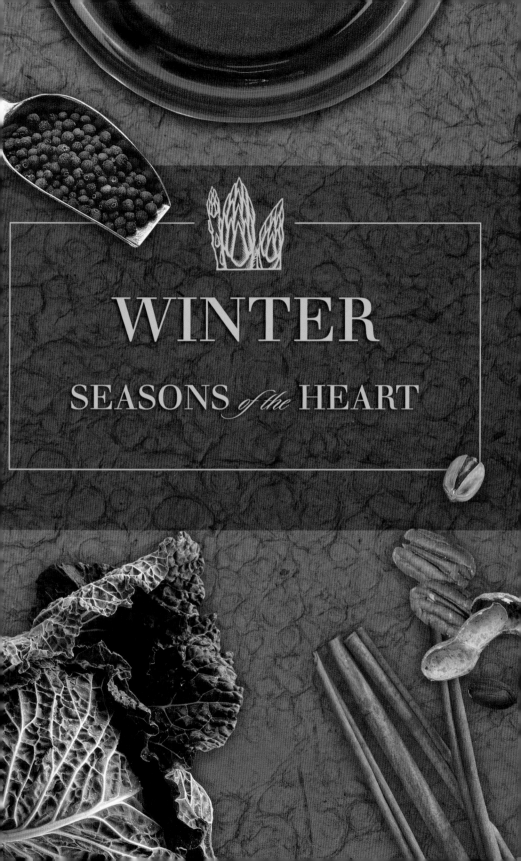

WINTER

SEASONS *of the* HEART

ITALIAN DIP

Number of Servings: 24

8 oz	Light mozzarella cheese, shredded	**1 c**	Artichoke hearts, drained and chopped
8 oz	Fat free cream cheese	**8 oz**	Red roasted peppers, drained and chopped
1/3 c	Light mayonnaise		
1 tsp	Minced garlic		
1/2 c	Sun dried tomatoes, chopped		

Preheat oven to 350°. Mix cream cheese, mozzarella cheese, mayonnaise and garlic in medium bowl until well blended. Spoon into 9-inch pie plate. Bake 10 minutes. Stir. Arrange tomatoes, artichokes and peppers on top of cheese mixture in 3 separate sections. Bake an additional 10 minutes. Serve with whole grain crackers.

Nutrition Facts

Serving Size 2 tablespoons (37g)
Servings Per Container 24

Amount Per Serving

Calories 60   Calories from Fat 20

	% Daily Value
Total Fat 2g	3%
Saturated Fat 1g	5%
Trans Fat 0g	
Cholesterol 5mg	2%
Sodium 240mg	10%
Total Carbohydrate 4g	1%
Dietary Fiber 0g	0%
Sugars 0g	
Protein 5g	

Artichokes are nutrient dense. For the 25 calories in a medium artichoke, you're getting 16 essential nutrients!

STUFFED MUSHROOMS

Number of Servings: 20

20	Medium mushrooms
3 Tbs	Trans fat free margarine
2 Tbs	White onion, chopped
3 Tbs	Red bell peppers, chopped
1/2 c	Whole wheat crackers, crushed
2 Tbs	Parmesan cheese, grated
1/2 tsp	Italian blend seasoning

Preheat oven to 400°. Remove stems from mushrooms. Finely chop enough of the stems to measure 1/4 cup; set aside. Cover and refrigerate remaining stems for other use. Melt margarine in large skillet on medium heat. Add 1/4 cup chopped mushroom stems, onions and peppers; cook and stir until vegetables are tender. Stir in cracker crumbs, cheese and Italian seasoning. Spoon crumb mixture evenly into mushroom caps. Place on ungreased baking sheet. Bake 15 minutes or until heated through.

Nutrition Facts

Serving Size 1 mushroom (25g)
Servings Per Container 20

Amount Per Serving

Calories 30 Calories from Fat 20

	% Daily Value
Total Fat 2g	3%
Saturated Fat 0.5g	3%
Trans Fat 0g	
Cholesterol 0mg	0%
Sodium 35mg	1%
Total Carbohydrate 2g	1%
Dietary Fiber 1g	4%
Sugars 0g	
Protein 1g	

SLOW-COOKED BLACK BEAN CHILI

Number of Servings: 10

1 lb	Boneless skinless chicken breasts, cubed	**1**	Red bell pepper
16 oz	Thick n' chunky salsa	**1 c**	White onion, chopped
3	15 oz cans black beans, drained and rinsed	**1 tsp**	Ground cumin seeds
		2 tsp	Chili pepper powder
1/2 c	Fat free reduced sodium chicken broth	**1 tsp**	Dried oregano
		1/4 c	Fat free sour cream

In a slow cooker, combine chicken, salsa, beans, broth, bell pepper, onion, cumin, chili powder and oregano. Cook on low setting 8 hours or until chicken is tender. Add water if mixture is thick. Serve with sour cream.

Nutrition Facts

Serving Size 1 cup (262g)
Servings Per Container 10

Amount Per Serving	
Calories 510	Calories from Fat 5

	% Daily Value
Total Fat 0.5g	1%
Saturated Fat 0g	0%
Trans Fat 0g	
Cholesterol 25mg	8%
Sodium 430mg	18%
Total Carbohydrate 86g	29%
Dietary Fiber 11g	44%
Sugars 14g	
Protein 36g	

Substitute beans for a meatless meal 2 to 4 times a week.

WINTER FRUIT SALAD

Number of Servings: 6

1/4 c	Sugar		**4 oz**	Low fat Swiss cheese, shredded
1/4 c	Fresh lemon juice		**1/2 c**	Pecans, chopped
2 tsp	White onion, chopped		**1/8 c**	Dried cranberries
1 tsp	Dijon mustard		**1/2 c**	Apples, cubed
1/2 tsp	Salt substitute		**1**	Pear, cubed
1/3 c	Canola oil			
1 Tbs	Poppy seed			
3 c	Romaine lettuce, chopped			

In a blender or food processor, combine sugar, lemon juice, onion, mustard and salt substitute. Process until well blended. With machine still running, add oil in a slow, steady stream until mixture is thick and smooth. Add poppy seeds and process just a few seconds more to mix. In a large serving bowl, combine the romaine lettuce, cheese, pecans, dried cranberries, apple and pear. Toss to mix, then pour dressing over salad just before serving and toss to coat.

Nutrition Facts

Serving Size 1 cup (132g)
Servings Per Container 6

Amount Per Serving

Calories 290 Calories from Fat 190

	% Daily Value
Total Fat 21g	**32%**
Saturated Fat 2g	10%
Trans Fat 0g	
Cholesterol 5mg	**2%**
Sodium 65mg	**3%**
Total Carbohydrate 20g	**7%**
Dietary Fiber 3g	12%
Sugars 15g	
Protein 7g	

WILTED SPINACH SALAD

Number of Servings: 2

2 1/2 c	Fresh baby spinach	**1 Tbs**	Sugar
2 Tbs	Green onions, tops and bulbs, chopped	**1 Tbs**	Cider vinegar
1	Red radish, sliced	**1 1/2 tsp**	Fresh lemon juice
1/8 tsp	Salt substitute	**1/2 tsp**	Cornstarch
1/8 tsp	Ground black pepper	**2 Tbs**	Water
2	Pieces of turkey bacon, crumbled	**1**	Hard boiled Omega-3 egg, chopped

In a salad bowl, combine the spinach, onion, radish, salt substitute and pepper; set aside.

In a small skillet, cook bacon over medium heat until crisp. Using a slotted spoon, remove to paper towels. Drain, reserving 1 tablespoon of the drippings. Combine the sugar, vinegar and lemon juice; stir into drippings. Cook and stir over low heat until sugar is dissolved. Combine cornstarch and water until smooth; add to skillet. Bring to a boil over medium heat; cook and stir for 1-2 minutes or until thickened.

Pour over spinach mixture and toss to coat. Top with crumbled bacon and egg.

Nutrition Facts

Serving Size 1 1/4 cups (129g)
Servings Per Container 2

Amount Per Serving

Calories 150   Calories from Fat 70

	% Daily Value
Total Fat 8g	12%
Saturated Fat 2g	10%
Trans Fat 0g	
Cholesterol 115mg	38%
Sodium 400mg	17%
Total Carbohydrate 12g	4%
Dietary Fiber 2g	8%
Sugars 8g	
Protein 8g	

SOUTHWEST LAYERED SALAD

Number of Servings: 6

6 c	Fresh romaine lettuce, chopped	**3/4 c**	Salsa
2 c	Dry black beans, cooked	**1/4 c**	Fat free ranch salad dressing
1 c	Frozen corn, thawed and drained	**8 oz**	Blue corn tortilla chips, broken
1/2 c	Reduced fat four cheese Mexican blend, finely shredded		

Arrange lettuce in bottom of glass serving bowl or on serving plate. Layer beans, corn, salsa and cheese evenly on top of lettuce. Drizzle with dressing. Break tortilla chips into small pieces; sprinkle to garnish.

Nutrition Facts

Serving Size 1 1/2 cups (237g)
Servings Per Container 6

Amount Per Serving

Calories 470   Calories from Fat 45

	% Daily Value
Total Fat 5g	8%
Saturated Fat 1g	5%
Trans Fat 0g	
Cholesterol 5mg	2%
Sodium 510mg	21%
Total Carbohydrate 85g	28%
Dietary Fiber 10g	40%
Sugars 9g	
Protein 21g	

Dried beans should be soaked and rinsed, then cooked in fresh water. This softens them, which reduces cooking time and dissolves some of the gas producing compounds which make the beans easier to digest.

CHICKEN, AVOCADO & BLACK BEAN SALAD

Number of Servings: 2

1/2 Tbs	Fresh lime juice	**1/4 tsp**	Ground black pepper
2 tsp	Extra virgin olive oil	**3 oz**	Grilled chicken breast strips, cubed
1 c	50% less salt black beans	**1/2 c**	Fresh avocado, cubed
2 Tbs	Red bell pepper, chopped	**6**	Cherry tomatoes
1/2 tsp	Minced garlic	**3/4 tsp**	Fresh cilantro
1/4 tsp	Crushed red chili pepper flakes		

Place lime juice in a large bowl and gradually whisk in olive oil. Stir in the beans, bell pepper, garlic, pepper flakes and pepper. Add chicken strips, avocado, cherry tomatoes and top with cilantro. Mix well.

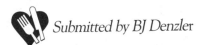 *Submitted by BJ Denzler*

Nutrition Facts

Serving Size 1 cup (264g)
Servings Per Container 2

Amount Per Serving

Calories 230 Calories from Fat 100

	% Daily Value
Total Fat 11g	17%
Saturated Fat 1.5g	8%
Trans Fat 0g	
Cholesterol 20mg	7%
Sodium 440mg	18%
Total Carbohydrate 22g	7%
Dietary Fiber 9g	36%
Sugars 3g	
Protein 15g	

OATMEAL PANCAKE

Number of Servings: 2

1/2 c	Old fashioned oats	**1/4 c**	1% cottage cheese
4	Egg whites	**1/4 tsp**	Ground cinnamon
1 tsp	Vanilla extract	**1/4 tsp**	Ground nutmeg

Process the oatmeal, cottage cheese, egg whites, vanilla extract, cinnamon and nutmeg in a blender until smooth. In a nonstick skillet, add the batter and cook over medium heat until both sides are lightly browned. You can top the pancake with a low sugar syrup of your choice. (Optional: top with fresh fruit).

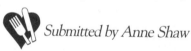 *Submitted by Anne Shaw*

Nutrition Facts

Serving Size 1 pancake (156g)
Servings Per Container 2

Amount Per Serving	
Calories 100 Calories from Fat 10	
	% Daily Value
Total Fat 1g	2%
Saturated Fat 0g	0%
Trans Fat 0g	
Cholesterol 0mg	0%
Sodium 230mg	10%
Total Carbohydrate 8g	3%
Dietary Fiber 1g	4%
Sugars 2g	
Protein 12g	

Rolled Oats: Oats that are steamed, pressed with a roller, then dried. Also known as old-fashioned oats. These will take about 15 minutes to cook.

Quick-cooking oats: Rolled oats that have been cut into smaller pieces and rolled thinner, thus they cook more quickly (about 5 minutes).

Instant oatmeal: Oatmeal that has been pre-cooked and dried. These days, instant oatmeal usually comes with flavor additives. Do not use in place of rolled or quick-cooking oatmeal.

Steel-cut oats or Scotch oats: Unrolled oats which have been cut into 2 or 3 pieces. Even with extended cooking time, they are quite chewy in texture. These are often used as a savory side dish.

TURKEY BREAKFAST SAUSAGE

Number of Servings: 8

1 lb 99% fat free ground turkey
3/4 tsp Salt substitute
1/2 tsp Sage

1/2 tsp Ground black pepper
1/4 tsp Ground ginger
1/4 tsp Chili pepper flakes

Crumble turkey into a large bowl. Add the salt substitute, sage, pepper, ginger and red pepper flakes; mix well. Shape into eight 2-inch patties. In a nonstick skillet, cook patties over medium heat for 6-8 minutes on each side or until no longer pink and a meat thermometer reads 165°.

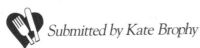 *Submitted by Kate Brophy*

Nutrition Facts

Serving Size 2-inch patty (57g)
Servings Per Container 8

Amount Per Serving	
Calories 60	Calories from Fat 5
	% Daily Value
Total Fat 1g	**2%**
Saturated Fat 0g	**0%**
Trans Fat 0g	
Cholesterol 20mg	**7%**
Sodium 35mg	**1%**
Total Carbohydrate 0g	**0%**
Dietary Fiber 0g	**0%**
Sugars 0g	
Protein 14g	

Substituting 99% lean ground turkey for ground beef reduces fat intake by approximately 75%.

QUICK & EASY
SALMON PATTIES

Number of Servings: 2

1	6 oz can, no salt added pink salmon, drained and rinsed
1	Hard boiled Omega-3 egg, chopped
1 Tbs	Whole wheat flour
2	Low sodium dill pickles, chopped

1 Tbs	Mustard
1 tsp	Original blend Mrs. Dash®
1/4 tsp	Ground black pepper
1/3	Onion, chopped

Preheat oven to 425°. Put salmon into a mixing bowl. Using a fork, break up the large pieces of salmon into smaller pieces. Add remaining ingredients and mix thoroughly. The mixture should be slightly moist. Add more whole wheat flour if needed to absorb any liquid that may stand in bottom of bowl. Form patties about 1/2-inch thick. Bake for 20 minutes or until golden brown.

Submitted by Jack King

Nutrition Facts

Serving Size 3 oz patty (281g)
Servings Per Container 2

Amount Per Serving	
Calories 330 Calories from Fat 160	
	% Daily Value
Total Fat 17g	26%
Saturated Fat 5g	25%
Trans Fat 0g	
Cholesterol 560mg	187%
Sodium 510mg	21%
Total Carbohydrate 7g	2%
Dietary Fiber 1g	4%
Sugars 2g	
Protein 33g	

Vitamin C is destroyed quickly in cooking – so cook your vitamin-rich vegetables in the smallest amount of water possible and for a short amount of time.

ORANGE ROUGHY ALMONDINE

Number of Servings: 2

1/4 c	Slivered almonds	**2 Tbs**	Lemon juice
12 oz	Orange roughy fillets	**1/8 tsp**	Hot pepper sauce
2 tsp	Light butter	**1/8 tsp**	Salt substitute
2 Tbs	Fat free reduced sodium chicken broth	**1/8 tsp**	Paprika

Place almonds in a small microwave-safe dish. Cover and microwave on high for 1-2 minutes or until lightly toasted.

Place the fillets (cod or haddock fillets can be substituted for orange roughy) in a 9-inch microwave-safe pie plate. Dot with light butter and sprinkle with almonds. Combine the remaining ingredients; pour over fillets. Cover and microwave at 70% power for 5 minutes or until fish flakes easily with a fork.

Nutrition Facts

Serving Size 5 oz fillet (217g)
Servings Per Container 2

Amount Per Serving

Calories 220   Calories from Fat 90

	% Daily Value
Total Fat 10g	15%
Saturated Fat 2g	10%
Trans Fat 0g	
Cholesterol 40mg	13%
Sodium 170mg	7%
Total Carbohydrate 4g	1%
Dietary Fiber 2g	8%
Sugars 1g	
Protein 28g	

TILAPIA WITH SAUTÉED VEGETABLES

Number of Servings: 4

2 Tbs	Original blend Mrs. Dash®	**1/4 c**	Yellow onion, chopped
1/4 tsp	Salt Substitute	**1 c**	Carrots, grated
1/4 tsp	Ground black pepper	**1**	Zucchini squash, sliced
2 tsp	Minced garlic	**1**	Butternut squash, peeled, chunked
1/2 c	Lemon juice	**2**	Roma tomatoes, sliced
1 1/2 lbs	Tilapia fillets		

Combine 1 tablespoon Mrs. Dash,® salt substitute, pepper, garlic and 1/4 cup lemon juice in small bowl; pour over fish. Grill, covered with grill lid, on a rack coated with cooking spray over medium heat 5-7 minutes or until fish flakes easily when tested with a fork.

Sauté onions, carrots, zucchini and squash in large skillet coated with cooking spray over medium heat 5-10 minutes or until tender. Stir in tomatoes, remaining Mrs. Dash® and remaining lemon juice. Serve fish immediately over vegetables.

Nutrition Facts

Serving Size 5-6 oz fillet (353g)
Servings Per Container 4

Amount Per Serving

Calories 230   Calories from Fat 30

	% Daily Value
Total Fat 3.5g	5%
Saturated Fat 1.5g	8%
Trans Fat 0g	
Cholesterol 160mg	53%
Sodium 270mg	11%
Total Carbohydrate 15g	5%
Dietary Fiber 3g	12%
Sugars 7g	
Protein 35g	

CRAB &
ASPARAGUS GRATIN

Number of Servings: 8

12 oz	Alaskan king crab legs	**1/8 tsp**	Ground nutmeg
10 oz	Frozen asparagus	**Dash**	Ground black pepper
1 Tbs	Trans fat free margarine	**1 c**	Skim milk
1 c	Fresh mushrooms, sliced	**2 Tbs**	Parmesan cheese, grated
1/4 c	White onion, chopped	**2 Tbs**	Almonds, sliced and toasted
1/8 tsp	Salt substitute		

Preheat oven to 400°. Thaw crab legs, if frozen. Remove meat from shells; cut meat into 1-inch pieces. Cook asparagus according to directions. Drain well and set aside. In a medium saucepan, melt margarine over medium heat. Add mushrooms and onion; cook until onion is tender. Stir in cornstarch, salt, nutmeg and pepper. Add milk all at once. Cook and stir until thickened and bubbly. Add crab and asparagus; continue to cook stirring for additional 5 minutes.

Nutrition Facts

Serving Size 1/2 cup (327g)
Servings Per Container 8

Amount Per Serving	
Calories 80	Calories from Fat 25

	% Daily Value
Total Fat 2.5g	4%
Saturated Fat 0.5g	3%
Trans Fat 0g	
Cholesterol 20mg	7%
Sodium 450mg	19%
Total Carbohydrate 4g	1%
Dietary Fiber 1g	4%
Sugars 2g	
Protein 11g	

In a small bowl, combine toasted almonds and parmesan cheese. Sprinkle over casserole. Bake for about 10 minutes or until mixture is heated through.

JEFFREY'S BLACKENED SWORDFISH

Number of Servings: 4

2 Tbs	Original blend Mrs. Dash®	**6 Tbs**	Ground black pepper
2 tsp	Cayenne pepper	**20 oz**	Swordfish steaks
		1 Tbs	Extra virgin olive oil

Preheat oven to 400°. Mix Mrs. Dash®, cayenne and black peppers together to make a rub. Rub steaks with olive oil and season both sides. In a skillet on high heat, pan sear 1 1/2 minutes each side of fish. After fish is seared, place fish in a 9x11-inch pan and put into oven for 3-5 minutes. Let sit for 5 minutes. Serve with Jeffrey's Sweet Potato Crab Hash (Winter, page 43) if desired.

Submitted by Jeffrey Wise

Nutrition Facts
Serving Size 5 oz fillet (125g)
Servings Per Container 4
Amount Per Serving
Calories 220　　Calories from Fat 80

	% Daily Value
Total Fat 9g	14%
Saturated Fat 2g	10%
Trans Fat 0g	
Cholesterol 50mg	17%
Sodium 125mg	5%
Total Carbohydrate 7g	2%
Dietary Fiber 3g	12%
Sugars 0g	
Protein 27g	

The preferred method for preparing fish is to bake, broil or grill.

JEFFREY'S SWEET POTATO CRAB HASH

Number of Servings: 8

4	Large sweet potatoes	**1 tsp**	Ground nutmeg
3 Tbs	Extra virgin olive oil	**3/4 c**	Green onions, tops and
1/2 tsp	Salt substitute		bulbs, chopped
1 tsp	Ground black pepper	**12 oz**	Dungeness crab

Preheat oven to 350°. Peel sweet potatoes; dice into 1/4-inch cubes. In a large bowl, measure olive oil, salt substitute, pepper and ground nutmeg. Stir to mix; then add sweet potatoes and stir to coat. On a baking sheet, evenly spread the potatoes to create a thin layer. Bake in oven for 4 minutes. Remove and set aside.

Nutrition Facts

Serving Size 1/2 cup (123g)
Servings Per Container 8

Amount Per Serving

Calories 150   Calories from Fat 50

	% Daily Value
Total Fat 6g	9%
Saturated Fat 1g	5%
Trans Fat 0g	
Cholesterol 30mg	10%
Sodium 190mg	8%
Total Carbohydrate 14g	5%
Dietary Fiber 2g	8%
Sugars 3g	
Protein 10g	

In a large skillet, sauté 1/4 cup green onions for 30 seconds. Add crab to skillet, mixing with onions for 1 to 1 1/2 minutes. Add potatoes to skillet and toss to blend well. Cook 5-10 minutes until potatoes are just done. Pour onto serving platter; garnish with remaining green onions and lemon wedges.

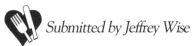 *Submitted by Jeffrey Wise*

COD WITH LEMON CREAM SAUCE

Number of Servings: 4

1 lb	Cod fillets		**1/2 c**	Skim milk
1 1/2 c	Water		**1 tsp**	Cornstarch
2 Tbs	Fresh lemon juice		**1/2 tsp**	Chicken bouillon
1/2 c	Carrots, chopped			dehydrated granules
1/2 c	Onions, chopped		**1/2 tsp**	Dill weed

Thaw fish, if frozen. Rinse and pat dry with paper towels. In a large skillet, combine water and lemon juice. Bring to a boil. Add fish. Simmer, covered, for 6-8 minutes or until fish flakes easily when tested with a fork. Remove fish and keep warm.

In a small covered saucepan, cook carrots and onions in a small amount of boiling water for 3-4 minutes or until crisp tender. Drain well. In a small bowl stir together milk, cornstarch, bouillon granules and dill. Add to vegetables in saucepan. Stir, cooking until thick and bubbly. Cook and stir for additional 2 minutes. Serve vegetable sauce over fish.

Nutrition Facts

Serving Size 4 oz fish filet with 1/4 cup sauce (278g)

Servings Per Container 4

Amount Per Serving

Calories 120   Calories from Fat 5

	% Daily Value
Total Fat 1g	2%
Saturated Fat 0g	0%
Trans Fat 0g	
Cholesterol 40mg	13%
Sodium 160mg	7%
Total Carbohydrate 7g	2%
Dietary Fiber 1g	4%
Sugars 3g	
Protein 22g	

SHRIMP DELIGHT

Number of Servings: 4

1 Tbs	Trans fat free margarine		**1 1/2 lbs**	Large shrimp, cooked
1 c	Mushrooms, sliced		**3 Tbs**	Fresh lemon juice
1/3 c	Celery, diced		**8**	Cherry tomatoes
1/4 c	Green onions, tops and bulbs, chopped		**1/8 tsp**	Ground black pepper
2 tsp	Minced garlic		**1 tsp**	Capers
1/4 c	Green bell peppers, chopped		**2 c**	Whole wheat vermicelli
2 Tbs	Fresh parsley, chopped			

Coat a large skillet with cooking spray; add margarine and place over medium-low heat until margarine is melted. Add next 6 ingredients to skillet; cover and cook 8-10 minutes or until vegetables are just tender, stirring occasionally. Peel and de-vein shrimp; add shrimp and lemon juice to cooked vegetables. Cook, uncovered, over medium-high heat 4-5 minutes or until shrimp are done. Stir in tomatoes, pepper and capers, if desired; cook 1 minute or until mixture is thoroughly heated. Serve over vermicelli. Garnish with celery leaves and lemon rind curl, if desired. (Optional: Use soy vermicelli.)

Nutrition Facts

Serving Size 1 cup (296g)
Servings Per Container 4

Amount Per Serving	
Calories 410	Calories from Fat 35

	% Daily Value
Total Fat 4g	6%
Saturated Fat 1g	5%
Trans Fat 0g	
Cholesterol 250mg	83%
Sodium 350mg	15%
Total Carbohydrate 62g	21%
Dietary Fiber 4g	16%
Sugars 15g	
Protein 28g	

SHEPHERD'S PIE

Number of Servings: 6

1	15 oz can black beans, drained and rinsed	**1 lb**	Red potatoes, peeled and cooked
1 c	No salt added tomato sauce	**1/2 c**	Reduced fat mozzarella cheese, shredded
2 Tbs	No salt added tomato paste	**2 Tbs**	Fat free sour cream
1 c	Yellow onion, chopped	**1 Tbs**	Trans fat free margarine
1/4 tsp	Dried oregano	**3/4 tsp**	Salt substitute
1/4 c	Water	**1/4 tsp**	Ground black pepper

Preheat oven to 350°. In a medium-size saucepan, stir together beans, tomato sauce and paste, onion, oregano, water, 1/4 teaspoon salt substitute and pepper. Bring to a boil over medium heat. Reduce heat, cover and simmer 20 minutes, or until liquid is thickened and onions are translucent. Spread the mixture into a shallow 1 1/2 quart casserole and set aside to cool. Mash potatoes and place in large bowl. Add mozzarella, sour cream, margarine and remaining 1/2 teaspoon salt substitute; beat until well blended. With a fork, spread potato topping over pie. Bake 45 minutes or until topping is bubbly and golden.

Nutrition Facts

Serving Size 1 cup (241g)
Servings Per Container 6

Amount Per Serving

Calories 180   Calories from Fat 35

% Daily Value

Total Fat 4g	6%
Saturated Fat 1.5g	8%
Trans Fat 0g	
Cholesterol 5mg	2%
Sodium 440mg	18%
Total Carbohydrate 26g	9%
Dietary Fiber 6g	24%
Sugars 4g	
Protein 9g	

CLASSIC MACARONI & CHEESE

Number of Servings: 8

2 c Whole wheat macaroni
1/2 c White onion, chopped
1/2 c Evaporated skim milk

1 Omega-3 egg
1/4 tsp Ground black pepper
1 1/4 c 2% reduced fat cheddar cheese, shredded

Preheat oven to 350°. Cook macaroni according to directions. Drain and set aside. Spray a casserole dish with nonstick cooking spray. Lightly spray sauté pan with nonstick cooking spray and add onions to saucepan; sauté for about 3 minutes.

In another bowl, combine macaroni, onions and remaining ingredients and mix thoroughly. Transfer mixture into casserole dish. Bake for 25 minutes or until bubbly. Let stand 10 minutes before serving.

Nutrition Facts	
Serving Size 1/2 cup (76g)	
Servings Per Container 8	
Amount Per Serving	
Calories 410 Calories from Fat 40	
	% Daily Value
Total Fat 4.5g	7%
Saturated Fat 2.5g	5%
Trans Fat 0g	
Cholesterol 35mg	12%
Sodium 170mg	7%
Total Carbohydrate 23g	8%
Dietary Fiber 2g	8%
Sugars 2g	
Protein 10g	

Always use 2% or light cheeses when cooking to reduce saturated fat but retain creaminess.

ROBERT'S EASY CASSEROLE

Number of Servings: 6

12 oz	Boneless skinless chicken breasts, cooked	**1**	14 oz can no salt added diced tomatoes
16 oz	Whole wheat pasta, cooked	**1 c**	Frozen spinach
1	10 3/4 oz can 98% fat free 30% reduced sodium cream of mushroom soup	**3/4 c**	2% reduced fat sharp cheddar cheese, shredded
		3/4 c	Water
		3/4 c	Low sodium whole wheat crackers

Preheat oven to 350°. In a casserole dish, combine the cooked chicken, soup, tomatoes, spinach, cheese and water until soup is not lumpy. Stir in the noodles until all is mixed evenly. Crush whole wheat crackers and sprinkle on top of mixture. Cook for 20 minutes.

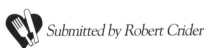 *Submitted by Robert Crider*

Nutrition Facts	
Serving Size 3/4 (338g)	
Servings Per Container 6	
Amount Per Serving	
Calories 480　　Calories from Fat 90	
	% Daily Value
Total Fat 10g	15%
Saturated Fat 2.5g	13%
Trans Fat 0g	
Cholesterol 120mg	40%
Sodium 490mg	20%
Total Carbohydrate 65g	22%
Dietary Fiber 9g	36%
Sugars 3g	
Protein 33g	

SESAME CHICKEN EDAMAME BOWL

Number of Servings: 6

2 tsp	Canola oil	**2 Tbs**	Low sodium soy sauce
1 Tbs	Fresh ginger root, grated	**1 Tbs**	Mirin wine
2 tsp	Minced garlic	**1 tsp**	Sesame oil
1 lb	Boneless skinless chicken breasts, cubed	**1/4 tsp**	Cornstarch
2 c	Shelled soybeans (edamame)	**1/2 c**	Green onions, tops and bulbs, chopped
2 c	Frozen mixed stir fry Chinese vegetables	**2 tsp**	Sesame seeds
		1/2 tsp	Salt substitute
		2 c	Brown rice, cooked

Heat canola oil in a large nonstick skillet over medium-high heat. Add ginger and garlic; sauté 1 minute or just until mixture begins to brown. Add chicken; sauté 2 minutes. Add edamame and stir-fry mix; sauté 3 minutes. Combine soy sauce, Mirin, sesame oil and cornstarch with a whisk. Add to pan; cook 1 minute. Remove from heat. Stir in onions, sesame seeds and salt substitute. Serve over rice.

Nutrition Facts

Serving Size 2/3 cup chicken and 1/3 cup rice (241g)
Servings Per Container 6

Amount Per Serving

Calories 270   Calories from Fat 60

	% Daily Value
Total Fat 6g	9%
Saturated Fat 0.5g	3%
Trans Fat 0g	
Cholesterol 45mg	15%
Sodium 260mg	11%
Total Carbohydrate 26g	9%
Dietary Fiber 5g	20%
Sugars 2g	
Protein 26g	

LAURA'S CHICKEN IN WINE

Number of Servings: 4

2 1/2 lbs	Boneless skinless chicken breasts
1/2 tsp	Salt substitute
1/2 tsp	Ground black pepper
5 oz	98% fat free 30% reduced sodium cream of mushroom soup
1/2 tsp	Ground oregano
1	Can, sliced mushrooms, drained
3/4 c	Dry white wine
1/4 tsp	Celery salt

Preheat oven to 350°. Place chicken in a medium dish; add salt substitute and pepper. In a small bowl, mix soup, mushrooms, wine and spices. Pour over chicken. Bake for 1-1 1/4 hours or until chicken is tender. Serve over brown or wild rice.

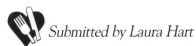

Submitted by Laura Hart

Nutrition Facts

Serving Size 4 oz breast plus 1/3 cup sauce (224g)
Servings Per Container 4

Amount Per Serving

Calories 200	Calories from Fat 20
	% Daily Value
Total Fat 2g	3%
Saturated Fat 0.5g	3%
Trans Fat 0g	
Cholesterol 85mg	28%
Sodium 220mg	9%
Total Carbohydrate 2g	1%
Dietary Fiber 0g	0%
Sugars 0g	
Protein 33g	

KATHY'S SPAGHETTI CASSEROLE

Number of Servings: 8

1 pkg	Whole wheat spaghetti	**2 c**	1% cottage cheese
2 c	No salt added tomato sauce	**1 c**	Fat free mozzarella cheese, shredded
1 c	2% reduced fat sharp cheddar cheese, shredded	**1 c**	98% fat free 30% reduced sodium cream of mushroom soup

Preheat oven to 350°. In a 9x13-inch pan, layer ingredients as follows: spaghetti, sauce (save some for topping), cheddar cheese, cottage cheese, mozzarella cheese, cream of mushroom soup and the rest of the sauce. Bake for one hour.

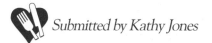 *Submitted by Kathy Jones*

Nutrition Facts

Serving Size 1 cup (205g)
Servings Per Container 8

Amount Per Serving

Calories 230   Calories from Fat 40

	% Daily Value
Total Fat 4.5g	7%
Saturated Fat 2g	10%
Trans Fat 0g	
Cholesterol 15mg	5%
Sodium 500mg	21%
Total Carbohydrate 29g	10%
Dietary Fiber 2g	8%
Sugars 3g	
Protein 19g	

CHICKEN TETRAZZINI

Number of Servings: 6

1/2 Tbs	Unsalted butter	**1/2 c**	Parmesan cheese, grated
1/2 c	White onion, chopped	**1/2**	Slice whole wheat bread
1/3 c	Celery, diced	**1/2 lb**	Whole wheat Vermicelli pasta, cooked and drained
1/2 tsp	Ground black pepper		
1/2 tsp	Salt substitute		
12 oz	Fresh mushrooms, sliced	**1/4 c**	Low fat cream cheese
1/4 c	Dry white wine	**1/3 c**	All purpose flour
10 oz	Fat free reduced sodium chicken broth	**3/4 lb**	Boneless skinless chicken breasts, cooked and chopped
1 c	Water		

Preheat oven to 350°. Melt butter in a large stockpot coated with cooking spray over medium-high heat. Add onion, celery, pepper, salt substitute and mushrooms, and sauté 4 minutes or until mushrooms are tender. Add wine; cook 1 minute.

Lightly spoon flour into a measuring cup; level with a knife. Gradually add flour to pan; cook 3 minutes, stirring constantly with a whisk (mixture will be thick). Gradually add broth and water, stirring constantly. Bring to a boil. Reduce heat, simmer 5 minutes, stirring frequently. Remove from heat.

Add 1/4 cup parmesan cheese and cream cheese. Add pasta and chicken and stir until blended. Place bread in a food processor; pulse 10 times or until coarse crumbs form. Combine bread crumbs and 1/4 cup parmesan cheese, sprinkle evenly over pasta mixture. Bake for 30 minutes or until lightly browned. Remove from oven; let stand 15 minutes.

Nutrition Facts

Serving Size 1 1/3 cups (295g)
Servings Per Container 6

Amount Per Serving	
Calories 310	Calories from Fat 50

	% Daily Value
Total Fat 6g	9%
Saturated Fat 3g	15%
Trans Fat 0g	
Cholesterol 45mg	15%
Sodium 390mg	16%
Total Carbohydrate 39g	13%
Dietary Fiber 2g	8%
Sugars 4g	
Protein 26g	

To prevent onion slices or wedges from falling through the grill rack, cut a large onion into 1/2-inch-thick slices or inch-wide wedges, then push a small metal or water-soaked bamboo skewer through the onion sections to secure them.

PARMESAN CHICKEN

Number of Servings: 4

1/4 c	All purpose flour	**12 oz**	Boneless skinless
1/2 tsp	Salt substitute		chicken breasts
1/2 tsp	Garlic powder	**1 Tbs**	Extra virgin olive oil
1	Omega-3 egg	**2 tsp**	Fresh lemon juice
1/3 c	Parmesan cheese, shredded		

Preheat oven to 350°. In a shallow bowl, combine the flour, salt substitute and garlic powder. In another bowl, beat the egg. Place the parmesan cheese in a third bowl. Coat chicken in flour mixture, then dip in the egg and roll in cheese.

In a skillet, brown chicken in oil on both sides. Transfer to a shallow 1-qt baking dish coated with nonstick cooking spray; drizzle with lemon juice. Bake, uncovered, for 18-20 minutes.

Nutrition Facts

Serving Size 3 oz breast (121g)
Servings Per Container 4

Amount Per Serving

Calories 200   Calories from Fat 70

	% Daily Value
Total Fat 8g	12%
Saturated Fat 2.5g	13%
Trans Fat 0g	
Cholesterol 100mg	33%
Sodium 200mg	8%
Total Carbohydrate 6g	2%
Dietary Fiber 0g	0%
Sugars 1g	
Protein 25g	

HEART HEALTHY PASTA SAUCE

Number of Servings: 12

30 oz	Marinara sauce	**1 tsp**	Garlic herb Mrs. Dash®
2 c	Soy buds	**1**	Clove garlic, chopped
1	Celery stalk, chopped	**1 tsp**	Salt substitute
3/4 c	Green onions, tops and bulbs, chopped	**8 oz**	Mushrooms, chopped
		3 c	Water

In a large heavy cooking pot, add marinara sauce, two cups of soy buds and three cups water. Add the remaining ingredients; mix well and simmer for several hours.

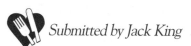 *Submitted by Jack King*

Nutrition Facts

Serving Size 1/2 C (198g)
Servings Per Container 12

Amount Per Serving

Calories 160   Calories from Fat 25

	% Daily Value
Total Fat 2.5g	4%
Saturated Fat 0g	0%
Trans Fat 0g	
Cholesterol 0mg	0%
Sodium 300mg	13%
Total Carbohydrate 17g	6%
Dietary Fiber 8g	32%
Sugars 1g	
Protein 23g	

Regular exercise is essential for weight management. Dieting alone will not lead to consistent and maintained weight loss. Both are needed for "balancing life."

CHICKEN SCALLOPINI WITH HERB SALAD

Number of Servings: 6

1 1/2 lbs	Boneless skinless chicken breasts		**1 oz**	Fresh watercress sprigs
1 c	1% buttermilk		**1/3 c**	Fresh parsley, chopped
1/2 tsp	Salt substitute		**1 Tbs**	Ground chives
1/2 c	All purpose flour		**2 Tbs**	Fresh shallots, chopped
2 tsp	Tarragon		**2 Tbs**	Lemon juice
1/2 tsp	Ground black pepper		**2 Tbs**	Extra virgin olive oil
1 Tbs	Canola oil		**1 Tbs**	Champagne vinegar
2 1/2 c	Frozen French cut green beans		**1 tsp**	Dijon mustard
4 c	Fresh baby spinach		**1/4 tsp**	Salt substitute
1 oz	Fresh arugula leaves		**1/8 tsp**	Ground black pepper

To prepare chicken, place each breast between 2 sheets of heavy-duty plastic wrap; pound each piece to 1/2-inch thickness using a meat mallet or rolling pin. Combine chicken and buttermilk in a large zip-top plastic bag; seal. Marinate in refrigerator for 2 hours, turning bag occasionally. Remove chicken from bag; discard marinade.

Pat chicken dry with paper towels; sprinkle with 1/2 teaspoon salt substitute. Combine flour, tarragon and 1/2 teaspoon black pepper in a shallow bowl. Dredge chicken in flour mixture; shake off excess. Heat oil in a large nonstick skillet over medium-high heat. Add chicken; cook 3 minutes on each side or until done.

To prepare salad, place French green beans into a large saucepan of boiling water; cook 3 minutes. Drain and plunge beans into ice water; drain.

CHICKEN SCALLOPINI
WITH HERB SALAD

continued

Place beans, spinach, arugula, watercress, parsley and chives in a large bowl. Combine shallots, juice, oil, vinegar, mustard, salt substitute and pepper in a small bowl, stirring with a whisk. Spoon 3 tablespoons shallot mixture over spinach mixture; toss gently to coat. Place 2 cups salad mixture onto each of 4 plates; top each serving with 1 chicken breast half. Drizzle chicken evenly with remaining shallot mixture.

Nutrition Facts

Serving Size 3 oz breast and 2 cups salad (284g)
Servings Per Container 6

Amount Per Serving

Calories 280   Calories from Fat 80

	% Daily Value
Total Fat 9g	14%
Saturated Fat 1.5g	8%
Trans Fat 0g	
Cholesterol 70mg	23%
Sodium 160mg	7%
Total Carbohydrate 19g	6%
Dietary Fiber 3g	12%
Sugars 5g	
Protein 31g	

CHICKEN & CHEDDAR RICE

Number of Servings: 4

1 lb	Boneless skinless chicken breasts
1 tsp	Garlic powder
10 3/4 oz	Skim milk (empty soup can)
1 1/2 c	Brown rice
2 c	Fresh broccoli florets, chopped

1 c	2% reduced fat cheddar cheese, shredded
1 can	98% fat free 30% reduced sodium cream of mushroom soup

Spray nonstick skillet with cooking spray. Add chicken; cover. Cook 15 minutes or until cooked through. Sprinkle with garlic powder. Add soup and milk. Bring to a boil. Stir in rice and broccoli; cover. Reduce heat to low; simmer 40 minutes or until rice is tender. Stir in 1/2 cup of the cheese; sprinkle with remaining cheese.

Nutrition Facts

Serving Size 1 cup (371g)
Servings Per Container 4

Amount Per Serving

Calories 380   Calories from Fat 70

	% Daily Value
Total Fat 8g	12%
Saturated Fat 3.5g	18%
Trans Fat 0g	
Cholesterol 85mg	28%
Sodium 420mg	18%
Total Carbohydrate 36g	12%
Dietary Fiber 3g	12%
Sugars 4g	
Protein 42g	

Pain is your body's way of telling you something is wrong. Don't ignore it.

CHICKEN & SAUSAGE JAMBALAYA

Number of Servings: 6

2 Tbs	Canola oil	**1/2 tsp**	Ground thyme
6 oz	Turkey sausage	**1/4 tsp**	Ground black pepper
3 c	Red bell peppers, chopped	**1/8 tsp**	Ground red chili pepper
3 c	Yellow onion, chopped	**3 tsp**	Minced garlic
2 c	Celery, diced	**1/2 c**	No salt added tomato puree
2 Tbs	Whole dried bay leaves	**2 3/4 c**	Fat free reduced sodium chicken broth
1 lb	Boneless skinless chicken breasts, cubed	**1 1/2 c**	Brown basmati rice
1 tsp	Ground basil	**1 c**	Green onions, tops and bulbs, chopped
1 tsp	Ground oregano	**1**	Jalapeno pepper, sliced

Heat oil in a large Dutch oven over medium-high heat. Add sausage; cook about 8 minutes, stirring occasionally. Add bell pepper, onion, celery and bay leaves; cook until vegetables are golden brown (about 14 minutes), stirring occasionally. Add chicken and next 6 ingredients; cook 4 minutes, stirring occasionally. Add tomato puree; cook 2 minutes, stirring occasionally. Add broth; bring to a boil. Stir in rice. Cover, reduce heat and simmer 20 minutes. Discard bay leaves. Stir in green onions. Add jalapeno pepper, if desired.

Nutrition Facts

Serving Size 1 1/3 cups (487g)
Servings Per Container 6

Amount Per Serving	
Calories 410	Calories from Fat 90

	% Daily Value
Total Fat 10g	15%
Saturated Fat 1.5g	8%
Trans Fat 0g	
Cholesterol 65mg	22%
Sodium 470mg	20%
Total Carbohydrate 53g	18%
Dietary Fiber 7g	28%
Sugars 9g	
Protein 30g	

KATE'S PASTA RUSTICA

Number of Servings: 8

1 tsp	Extra virgin olive oil	**1/2 tsp**	Salt substitute
1/2 c	Yellow onion, chopped	**16 oz**	Whole wheat penne pasta
2 Tbs	Minced garlic	**28 oz**	Canned tomato puree
3/4 lb	Light turkey sausage	**1/4 c**	Fat free ricotta cheese
1 tsp	Fresh basil leaves, chopped	**1/2 c**	Fat free parmesan cheese
1 tsp	Fresh oregano	**16 oz**	Mozzarella soy cheese, shredded
1/4 tsp	Crushed chili pepper flakes		

Preheat oven to 350°. In a large Dutch oven, over medium heat, warm oil. Add onion and cook until golden brown, about 5 minutes. Add garlic and cook, stirring for 1 minute. Add sausage and cook, breaking up into bite-size pieces until no longer pink, about 6 minutes. Stir in basil, oregano, red pepper flakes and salt substitute. Add tomato puree and bring to a boil.

Reduce heat to medium low and simmer, stirring occasionally until thickened, about 10-12 minutes. Taste and adjust seasoning. Using cooking spray, lightly spray a 9x13-inch baking dish.

Bring a large pot 3/4 full of water to a boil over high heat. Add pasta, stir well and cook until barely al dente (tender but not firm to the bite), about

KATE'S PASTA RUSTICA

continued

10-12 minutes. Drain well. In a large bowl, toss pasta with sauce, ricotta and mozzarella. Spread in prepared baking dish and sprinkle with parmesan. Bake until cheeses are melted and tips of pasta are crusty, about 30-35 minutes. Let stand 5 minutes before serving.

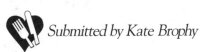 *Submitted by Kate Brophy*

Nutrition Facts

Serving Size 1 cup (283g)
Servings Per Container 8

Amount Per Serving

Calories 470 Calories from Fat 100

	% Daily Value
Total Fat 12g	18%
Saturated Fat 1g	5%
Trans Fat 0g	
Cholesterol 35mg	12%
Sodium 390mg	16%
Total Carbohydrate 53g	18%
Dietary Fiber 6g	24%
Sugars 4g	
Protein 33g	

TACO PORK SKILLET

Number of Servings: 4

2 Tbs	Fat free Italian salad dressing	**1 c**	Zucchini, sliced
1 lb	Lean pork tenderloin, cut into bite size pieces	**2 c**	Instant brown rice
1 pkg	Reduced sodium taco seasoning	**1/3 c**	2% reduced fat sharp cheddar cheese, shredded
1 c	Red bell peppers, sliced		
1 c	Green bell peppers, sliced		

Heat dressing in large skillet on medium-high heat. Add pork; sprinkle with half of the seasoning mix. Stir-fry 2 minutes. Add vegetables, rice, water and remaining seasoning mix; mix well. Bring mixture to a boil. Reduce heat to medium; cover. Simmer 5 minutes. Sprinkle with cheese; cover. Let stand 5 minutes.

Nutrition Facts

Serving Size 1 cup (249g)
Servings Per Container 4

Amount Per Serving

Calories 350   Calories from Fat 70

	% Daily Value
Total Fat 8g	12%
Saturated Fat 2.5g	13%
Trans Fat 0g	
Cholesterol 80mg	27%
Sodium 300mg	13%
Total Carbohydrate 39g	13%
Dietary Fiber 3g	12%
Sugars 3g	
Protein 31g	

DELICIOUS MEAT LOAF

Number of Servings: 6

1 lb	96% lean ground beef
1	6 oz can no salt added tomato paste
1/4 c	White onion, chopped
1/4 c	Green bell peppers, chopped
1/4 c	Red bell peppers, chopped
1 c	Red tomatoes, diced
1/2 tsp	Mustard
1/4 tsp	Ground black pepper
1/2 tsp	Green chili peppers, chopped
2 tsp	Minced garlic
2 Tbs	Green onions, tops and bulbs, chopped
1/2 tsp	Ground ginger
1/8 tsp	Ground nutmeg
1 tsp	Fresh orange peel, grated
1/4 tsp	Ground thyme
1/4 c	Plain bread crumbs

Preheat oven to 350°. Mix all ingredients together; blend well. Place in loaf pan (preferably a pan with a drip rack) and bake uncovered at 350° for 50 minutes. Uncover pan and continue baking for 12 minutes.

Nutrition Facts

Serving Size 1 1/4-inch slice (163g)
Servings Per Container 6

Amount Per Serving	
Calories 150 Calories from Fat 35	
	% Daily Value
Total Fat 3.5g	5%
Saturated Fat 1g	5%
Trans Fat 0g	
Cholesterol 40mg	13%
Sodium 115mg	5%
Total Carbohydrate 12g	4%
Dietary Fiber 2g	8%
Sugars 5g	
Protein 17g	

Use music to keep you entertained while exercising.

JAN'S HEART-Y HOME STYLE SWEET POTATOES

Number of Servings: 12

6 c	Sweet potatoes, peeled and cubed	**1/2 tsp**	Ground black pepper
2 Tbs	Extra virgin olive oil	**1 tsp**	Ground cinnamon
1/2 tsp	Light salt	**1 tsp**	Splenda®

Place sweet potato cubes in a glass dish with 1/2-inch water. Cover with plastic wrap. Steam sweet potatoes in the microwave on high for 4 minutes. Remove from microwave, drain and dry potatoes. Drizzle with olive oil. Sprinkle with salt and pepper to taste and bake in the oven on 400° until lightly crisp. Remove from oven and sprinkle with cinnamon and Splenda®.

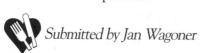 *Submitted by Jan Wagoner*

Nutrition Facts

Serving Size 1/2 cup (91g)
Servings Per Container 12

Amount Per Serving

Calories 110   Calories from Fat 20

	% Daily Value
Total Fat 2.5g	4%
Saturated Fat 0g	0%
Trans Fat 0g	
Cholesterol 0mg	0%
Sodium 55mg	2%
Total Carbohydrate 21g	7%
Dietary Fiber 2g	8%
Sugars 0g	
Protein 2g	

BAKED SWEET ONION

Number of Servings: 1

1 tsp Trans fat free margarine
1/4 tsp Garlic powder

1 Medium sweet onion, whole

Preheat oven to 350°. Slice whole onion 4-6 times starting at top of onion and cutting down 3/4 into the whole onion, creating a partially open bloom. Put onion into an oven safe dish. Spread margarine on top of onion. Sprinkle garlic powder on top of margarine. Bake for 10-15 minutes or until tender.

Nutrition Facts

Serving Size 1 onion (153g)
Servings Per Container 1

Amount Per Serving	
Calories 90	Calories from Fat 25

	% Daily Value
Total Fat 3g	5%
Saturated Fat 1g	5%
Trans Fat 0g	
Cholesterol 0mg	0%
Sodium 35mg	1%
Total Carbohydrate 15g	5%
Dietary Fiber 3g	12%
Sugars 9g	
Protein 2g	

There are many methods recommended for cutting onions to avoid tears. Use the one that works for you. You can: cut the root off last; refrigerate before cutting; peel them under cold water; have a fan behind you or alongside to blow the vapors away; place a piece of bread on the knife tip to absorb the fumes; chew gum while peeling and slicing onions, hold your breath and cut them as quickly as you can or have someone else cut them for you!

GARLIC BUTTER GREEN BEANS

Number of Servings: 4

1 lb	Fresh green beans		**1 Tbs**	Fresh lemon juice
1 tsp	Minced garlic		**1/2 tsp**	Sugar
1 Tbs	Salted light butter		**1/8 tsp**	Ground black pepper

Place beans in a steamer basket; place in a large saucepan over 1 inch of water. Bring to a boil; cover and steam for 7-9 minutes or until crisp-tender. Meanwhile, in a small nonstick saucepan, cook garlic and light butter until tender. Remove from the heat; stir in the lemon juice, sugar and pepper. Transfer the beans to a serving bowl; add garlic butter mixture and stir to coat.

Nutrition Facts

Serving Size 3/4 cup (123g)
Servings Per Container 4

Amount Per Serving

Calories 50   Calories from Fat 15

	% Daily Value
Total Fat 2g	3%
Saturated Fat 1g	5%
Trans Fat 0g	
Cholesterol 5mg	2%
Sodium 25mg	1%
Total Carbohydrate 9g	3%
Dietary Fiber 4g	16%
Sugars 2g	
Protein 2g	

MUFFINS

Number of Servings: 12

1 c	Dates, chopped	**3 1/2 c**	Old fashioned oats
1 Tbs	Baking powder	**3/4 c**	Skim milk
1 c	Sugar free orange marmalade jam	**2**	Omega-3 eggs
1 Tbs	Canola oil	**1 c**	Walnuts, chopped

Preheat oven to 375°. Mix oats, milk and marmalade and allow to stand at least 30 minutes. Add eggs, oil, baking powder, chopped dates and nuts to oats mixture, stirring after each addition until completely blended. Spray regular size muffin tins with canola oil. Fill tins even with top. Bake 20 minutes or until lightly brown. Remove from oven and cool about 15 minutes before removing from pan.

Substitute any kind of low sugar or sugar free jam for orange marmalade and any dried fruit for chopped dates.

Nutrition Facts

Serving Size 1 muffin (128g)
Servings Per Container 12

Amount Per Serving

Calories 280 Calories from Fat 120

	% Daily Value
Total Fat 13g	20%
Saturated Fat 2g	10%
Trans Fat 0g	
Cholesterol 170mg	57%
Sodium 170mg	7%
Total Carbohydrate 35g	12%
Dietary Fiber 4g	16%
Sugars 11g	
Protein 12g	

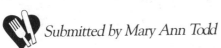 *Submitted by Mary Ann Todd*

LAYERED FRUIT SENSATION

Number of Servings: 16

1	Sugar free angel food cake
3 Tbs	Fresh orange juice
2 1/2 c	Skim milk
1	Small box sugar free instant vanilla pudding
1 1/2 c	Light whipped topping
2 1/2 c	Frozen mixed berries
1/4 tsp	Almond extract

Cut cake into cubes; place in large bowl. Combine orange juice and almond extract. Drizzle over cake cubes; toss lightly.

Pour milk into another large bowl. Add dry pudding mix. Beat with wire whisk 2 minutes or until well blended. Gently stir in 1 cup of the whipped topping.

Layer half the cake cubes in bottom of 2 quart glass serving bowl or 2 quart round baking dish. Reserve a few of the thawed berries for garnish. Add a layer with half of the berries. Add a layer of pudding mixture on top of berries. Repeat layers. Cover with plastic wrap. Refrigerate 2-6 hours before serving. Top with remaining 1/2 cup whipped topping and reserved berries just before serving.

Nutrition Facts

Serving Size 1/2 cup (86g)
Servings Per Container 16

Amount Per Serving

Calories 70	Calories from Fat 5
	% Daily Value
Total Fat 1g	2%
Saturated Fat 1g	5%
Trans Fat 0g	
Cholesterol 0mg	0%
Sodium 100mg	4%
Total Carbohydrate 12g	4%
Dietary Fiber 1g	4%
Sugars 4g	
Protein 3g	

OATMEAL RAISIN COOKIES

Number of Servings: 24

2 c	Whole wheat flour	1/2 c	Apple juice
2 c	Old fashioned oats	1/4 c	Unsweetened applesauce
2 tsp	Baking soda		
1/4 tsp	Ground nutmeg	2 tsp	Vanilla extract
1 3/4 tsp	Ground cinnamon	3/4 c	Seedless raisins
1/4 tsp	Ground allspice	3	Egg whites
3/4 c	Light honey		

Preheat oven to 350°. In a large bowl, combine flour, oats, baking soda, cinnamon, nutmeg and allspice; mix well. In a medium bowl, combine honey, apple juice, applesauce, vanilla, raisins and egg whites. Gently stir into flour mixture and mix until just blended. Do not over mix. Drop by heaping teaspoons onto nonstick cookie baking sheet. Lightly pat down each mound. Bake for 12 minutes. Allow cookies to cool slightly before removing from sheet.

Nutrition Facts

Serving Size 1 cookie (71g)
Servings Per Container 24

Amount Per Serving

Calories 130   Calories from Fat 5

% Daily Value

Total Fat 0.5g	1%
Saturated Fat 0g	0%
Trans Fat 0g	
Cholesterol 0mg	0%
Sodium 160mg	7%
Total Carbohydrate 25g	8%
Dietary Fiber 2g	8%
Sugars 13g	
Protein 6g	

CHOCOLATE ÉCLAIR CAKE

Number of Servings: 12

3 1/4 c	Skim milk	**1/3 c**	Unsweetened cocoa powder
2	Small boxes sugar free instant vanilla pudding	**1/4 c**	Trans fat free margarine
1 c	Fat free whipped topping	**1 tsp**	Vanilla extract
1/2 tsp	Salt substitute	**24**	Low fat graham cracker squares
1 c	Splenda®		

Line bottom of 9x13-inch pan with graham crackers. Mix pudding with 3 cups of milk until smooth. Set aside the remaining 1/4 cup milk. Fold fat free whipped topping into pudding mixture. Spread 1/2 of pudding mixture onto bottom layer of graham crackers. Top pudding with second layer of graham crackers. Pour rest of pudding mixture over crackers and top with a final layer of graham crackers.

Nutrition Facts

Serving Size 1/2 cup (111g)
Servings Per Container 12

Amount Per Serving	
Calories 160	Calories from Fat 35

	% Daily Value
Total Fat 4g	6%
Saturated Fat 1g	5%
Trans Fat 0g	
Cholesterol 0mg	0%
Sodium 190mg	8%
Total Carbohydrate 26g	9%
Dietary Fiber 1g	4%
Sugars 9g	
Protein 4g	

Icing: In a small saucepan, melt margarine. Stirring continuously, add salt, Splenda®, 1/4 cup milk and cocoa; heat throughout and bring to a boil for one minute. Remove from heat; add vanilla and stir until smooth. Allow to cool to slightly warm. Ice top layer of graham crackers with chocolate icing. Cover and refrigerate overnight or for several hours.

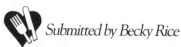

Submitted by Becky Rice

BANANA CRUNCH CAKE

Number of Servings: 8

3/4 c	Old fashioned oats	**1/4 c**	Splenda®
1/8 c	Brown sugar, packed	**3/4 c**	Banana, mashed
1/8 c	Splenda®	**2**	Omega-3 eggs
2 Tbs	Trans fat free margarine	**1 tsp**	Vanilla extract
2 Tbs	Walnuts, chopped	**1 oz**	Oat flour
1/2 Tbs	Ground cinnamon	**3/4 c**	Whole wheat flour
1/2 c	Trans fat free margarine	**1 tsp**	Salt substitute
1/4 c	Brown sugar, packed	**1 tsp**	Baking soda
		1/2 c	Walnuts, chopped

Preheat oven to 350°.

Crunch Topping: In a small bowl, combine first 6 ingredients; mix well. Set aside.

Cake: In a large bowl, combine brown sugar, Splenda® and margarine; beat until light and fluffy. Blend in banana, eggs and vanilla; mix well. In a medium bowl, combine flours, salt substitute and baking soda; add to wet mixture. Mix well. Stir in nuts. Pour into greased 8-inch square baking pan; sprinkle crunch topping evenly over batter. Bake 40-45 minutes or until wooden pick inserted in center comes out clean.

Nutrition Facts

Serving Size 2-inch square (96g)
Servings Per Container 8

Amount Per Serving	
Calories 350 Calories from Fat 200	
	% Daily Value
Total Fat 22g	34%
Saturated Fat 2.5g	13%
Trans Fat 0g	
Cholesterol 45mg	15%
Sodium 280mg	12%
Total Carbohydrate 33g	11%
Dietary Fiber 4g	16%
Sugars 13g	
Protein 6g	

CAPPUCCINO PUDDING CAKE

Number of Servings: 9

1 c	All purpose flour
1/4 c	Sugar
1/3 c	Splenda®
2 Tbs	Unsweetened cocoa powder
2 tsp	Baking powder
1/4 tsp	Salt substitute
1/2 c	Evaporated skim milk
1 tsp	Canola oil
1 tsp	Vanilla extract
1/8 c	Semi sweet chocolate chips
1/4 c	Unsweetened cocoa powder
1/4 c	Splenda® brown sugar blend
1 3/4 c	Hot water
1/4 c	Sugar free Swiss mocha instant coffee powder

Preheat oven to 350°. Spray pan with nonstick cooking spray. Combine first 6 ingredients in a 9-inch square baking pan; stir well. Stir in milk, oil and vanilla. Stir in chocolate chips. Combine Splenda® brown sugar blend and 1/4 cup cocoa; sprinkle over batter. Combine HOT water and coffee mix, stir to dissolve. Pour coffee mixture over batter (do not stir). Bake for 40 minutes or until cake springs back when lightly touched in center. Serve warm.

Nutrition Facts

Serving Size 1/2 cup (97g)
Servings Per Container 9

Amount Per Serving

Calories 130   Calories from Fat 15

	% Daily Value
Total Fat 1.5g	4%
Saturated Fat 0.5g	3%
Trans Fat 0g	
Cholesterol 0mg	0%
Sodium 140mg	6%
Total Carbohydrate 28g	9%
Dietary Fiber 1g	4%
Sugars 14g	
Protein 3g	

BROWNIES

Number of Servings: 10

1/2 c	Sugar		**2**	Omega-3 eggs
1/4 c	Splenda®		**1/4 c**	Light butter, unsalted
1/3 c	Splenda® brown sugar blend		**1/2 c**	Light cream cheese, softened
3 oz	Cocoa powder		**1/2 c**	Walnuts, chopped
1 tsp	Vanilla extract			

Mix together all ingredients in a bowl except walnuts. Pour into pie plate sprayed with nonstick cooking spray. Top with chopped walnuts. You can use a low fat crust if desired. Bake for 45 minutes.

Nutrition Facts

Serving Size 2-inch wedge (58g)
Servings Per Container 10

Amount Per Serving

Calories 180   Calories from Fat 90

	% Daily Value
Total Fat 10g	15%
Saturated Fat 4.5g	23%
Trans Fat 0g	
Cholesterol 50mg	17%
Sodium 60mg	3%
Total Carbohydrate 14g	5%
Dietary Fiber 3g	12%
Sugars 15g	
Protein 5g	

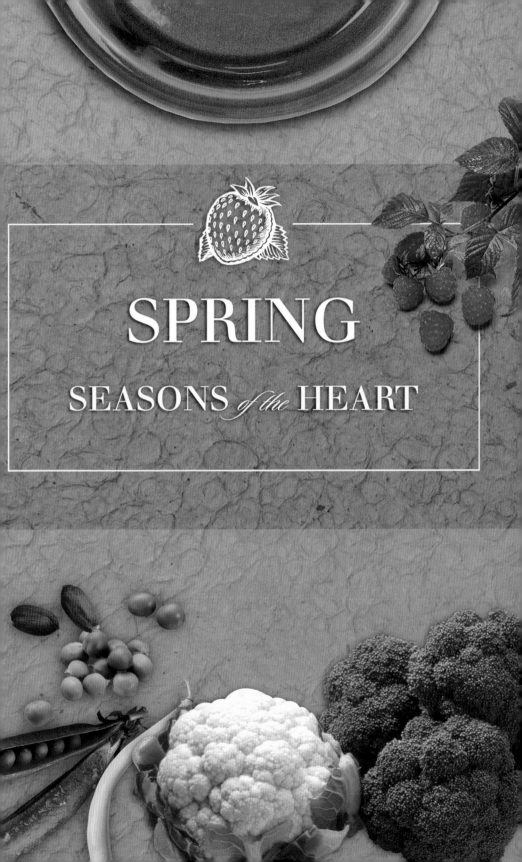

SPRING

SEASONS *of the* HEART

CHEESY ASPARAGUS BITES

Number of Servings: 60

1/2 c	White onion, chopped	**1/4 tsp**	Ground black pepper
1 tsp	Minced garlic	**1/4 tsp**	Oregano
2 Tbs	Extra virgin olive oil	**1/8 tsp**	Hot pepper sauce
2 c	2% reduced fat sharp cheddar cheese	**2**	Omega-3 eggs
1/4 c	Plain bread crumbs	**1/2 c**	Egg substitute
2 Tbs	Fresh parsley, chopped	**1 lb**	Fresh asparagus, 1/2-inch pieces

Rinse asparagus. Cut and discard the thick, rough ends. Then cut asparagus into 1/2-inch pieces and set aside.

Preheat oven to 350°.
In a skillet, sauté onion and garlic in oil until tender.
In a medium bowl, combine cheese, bread crumbs, parsley, pepper, oregano and hot pepper sauce. Stir in the cooked onion mixture and beaten eggs.
Stir in asparagus pieces.

Pour into a 9-inch square baking pan coated with nonstick cooking spray. Bake for 30 minutes or until knife inserted in the center comes out clean. Let stand for 15 minutes. Cut into small squares and serve slightly warm.

Nutrition Facts

Serving Size 1-inch square (17g)
Servings Per Container 60

Amount Per Serving	
Calories 20	Calories from Fat 15

	% Daily Value
Total Fat 1.5g	2%
Saturated Fat 0.5g	3%
Trans Fat 0g	
Cholesterol 10mg	3%
Sodium 40mg	2%
Total Carbohydrate 1g	0%
Dietary Fiber 0g	0%
Sugars 0g	
Protein 2g	

BRUSCHETTA POMADORO

Number of Servings: 12

6	Garlic cloves	**1/2 Tbs**	Ground black pepper
12	Mini sourdough baguette pieces	**8**	Plum tomatoes
2 Tbs	Extra virgin olive oil	**1 tsp**	Fresh basil leaves, chopped (or oregano)

Preheat broiler or a charcoal fire. Mash the garlic cloves with a heavy knife handle, crushing them just enough to split them to loosen the peel; discard peel. Cut tomatoes in half lengthwise; using the tip of a paring knife pick out all the seeds you can. Dice the tomatoes into 1/2-inch cubes. Wash the basil leaves, shake them thoroughly dry and tear them into small pieces (omit this step if using oregano).

Nutrition Facts

Serving Size 1 piece (102g)
Servings Per Container 12

Amount Per Serving

Calories 170   Calories from Fat 25

	% Daily Value
Total Fat 3g	5%
Saturated Fat 0g	0%
Trans Fat 0g	
Cholesterol 0mg	0%
Sodium 330mg	14%
Total Carbohydrate 31g	10%
Dietary Fiber 2g	8%
Sugars 2g	
Protein 5g	

Grill the bread to a golden brown on both sides. As the bread comes off the grill, while it is still hot, rub one side of each slice with the mashed garlic and top it with diced tomato, sprinkle with basil or oregano, add pepper and lightly drizzle each slice with olive oil. Serve warm.

MARY'S CHICKEN AND ASPARAGUS SOUP

Number of Servings: 8

28 oz	Fat free reduced sodium chicken broth
1/2 c	White wine
1 c	Water
8 oz	Fresh asparagus
1 c	Fresh mushrooms
1/4 c	Green onions, tops and bulbs, minced
1 Tbs	Cornstarch
1/4 c	Water
1/2 tsp	Minced garlic
1/2 tsp	Salt substitute
1/2 tsp	Ground black pepper
12 oz	Boneless skinless chicken breasts, cooked, cubed

Combine the above ingredients except chicken and simmer. When asparagus becomes tender, add chicken breast. Heat thoroughly on medium heat. In a small bowl, combine cornstarch with 1/4 cup water. Stir in cornstarch mixture after soup begins to boil. Reduce heat to low. When broth is slightly thickened, add onion and remove from heat.

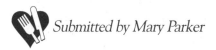 *Submitted by Mary Parker*

Nutrition Facts

Serving Size 1 cup (235g)
Servings Per Container 8

Amount Per Serving

Calories 70   Calories from Fat 5

	% Daily Value
Total Fat 0.5g	1%
Saturated Fat 0g	0%
Trans Fat 0g	
Cholesterol 25mg	8%
Sodium 250mg	10%
Total Carbohydrate 3g	1%
Dietary Fiber 1g	4%
Sugars 1g	
Protein 11g	

When cooking a dish with both vegetables and meat (i.e., stir frys and stews), reduce the amount of meat by 1/3 and increase the amount of vegetables by 1/3. You will hardly notice!

AUNT HILDA'S BROCCOLI SALAD

Number of Servings: 8

4 c Fresh broccoli florets, chopped
1 c 2% reduced fat cheddar cheese, shredded
1 Omega-3 egg, hard boiled, chopped
1 Egg white, hard boiled, chopped

1/2 c Celery, diced
1/4 c Low sodium pickles, chopped
1/4 c Red onion, diced
1/4 c Fat free mayonnaise

Line large bowl with leaf lettuce. Combine all ingredients in a bowl and chill. (Optional: 1/2 cup sliced green olives with pimentos can be added. However, it will increase sodium content by 80 mg. per serving).

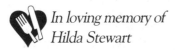 *In loving memory of Hilda Stewart*

Nutrition Facts		
Serving Size 1/2 cup (105g)		
Servings Per Container 8		
Amount Per Serving		
Calories 60	Calories from Fat 15	
		% Daily Value
Total Fat 2g		3%
Saturated Fat 1g		5%
Trans Fat 0g		
Cholesterol 25mg		8%
Sodium 170mg		7%
Total Carbohydrate 5g		2%
Dietary Fiber 1g		4%
Sugars 1g		
Protein 6g		

CHICKEN STRAWBERRY SPINACH SALAD

Number of Servings: 2

3/4 lb	Boneless skinless chicken breasts	**2 c**	Fresh baby spinach
1/4 c	Fat free reduced sodium chicken broth	**1 c**	Romaine lettuce
1/4 c	Poppy seed salad dressing	**1 c**	Strawberries, sliced
		1/4 c	Almonds, sliced

Place chicken on a double thickness of heavy duty foil. Combine chicken broth and 1 tablespoon of poppy seed dressing; spoon over chicken. Fold edges of foil around chicken mixture, leaving center open. Grill, covered, over medium heat for 10-12 minutes or until chicken juices run clear.

Nutrition Facts

Serving Size 1 cup (366g)
Servings Per Container 2

Amount Per Serving

Calories 450 Calories from Fat 180

	% Daily Value
Total Fat 20g	31%
Saturated Fat 2.5g	13%
Trans Fat 0g	
Cholesterol 110mg	37%
Sodium 410mg	17%
Total Carbohydrate 20g	7%
Dietary Fiber 4g	16%
Sugars 11g	
Protein 43g	

In a salad bowl, combine the spinach, torn romaine and strawberries. Add the chicken and remaining poppy seed dressing; toss to coat. Sprinkle with toasted almonds.

OATMEAL WITH APPLES AND WALNUTS

Number of Servings: 6

1/4 c Walnuts, chopped
3 c Skim milk
1-1/2 c Old fashioned oats
1 Granny Smith apple
1/2 tsp Ground cinnamon

1/4 tsp Salt substitute
1/2 tsp Vanilla extract
3 Tbs Brown sugar
 Splenda® blend
3 Tbs Slivered almonds

Combine milk and next 4 ingredients in a medium saucepan. Bring to a boil over medium heat. Stir in vanilla. Cover, reduce heat and simmer 5 minutes or until thick. Sprinkle with walnuts, brown sugar and almonds.

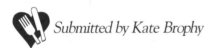 *Submitted by Kate Brophy*

Nutrition Facts

Serving Size 2/3 cup (183g)
Servings Per Container 6

Amount Per Serving	
Calories 210	Calories from Fat 60

	% Daily Value
Total Fat 6g	9%
Saturated Fat 0.5g	3%
Trans Fat 0g	
Cholesterol 0mg	0%
Sodium 65mg	3%
Total Carbohydrate 24g	8%
Dietary Fiber 3g	12%
Sugars 15g	
Protein 9g	

To reduce fat content, substitute applesauce for 1/2 the amount of fat in original recipe. Or, use all applesauce to produce a low calorie, moist product.

ZIPLOC® OMELET

Number of Servings: 1

1 Omega-3 egg   **1** Egg white

Please follow the instructions precisely. Have guests write their name with permanent marker on a quart size freezer bag. Crack open the Omega-3 egg and add to plastic bag along with an egg white from a regular egg; shake to combine them. Have a variety of ingredients to add to the bag, such as low fat cheeses, turkey and lean ham pieces, mushrooms, tomatoes, peppers, onions, etc.

Nutrition Facts	
Serving Size 1 bagged omelet (83g)	
Servings Per Container 1	
Amount Per Serving	
Calories 90	Calories from Fat 35
	% Daily Value
Total Fat 4g	6%
Saturated Fat 1g	5%
Trans Fat 0g	
Cholesterol 180mg	60%
Sodium 55mg	2%
Total Carbohydrate 0g	0%
Dietary Fiber 0g	0%
Sugars 0g	
Protein 10g	

Have each guest add the prepared ingredients to the bag and shake. Get all the AIR out of the bag and zip it up. Place the bags into rolling, boiling water for exactly 13 minutes. Usually 6-8 bags will fit in a large pot. Open the bags and the omelet will roll out easily. Serve with fresh fruit.

PENNY'S SALMON WITH BLACK BEAN SALSA

Number of Servings: 4

1 lb	Fresh wild Alaskan salmon fillets	**1/4 c**	Fresh cilantro
1/4 tsp	Salt substitute	**2 Tbs**	Jalapeno peppers, diced
1/4 tsp	Ground black pepper	**1/2 tsp**	Minced garlic
1 c	Black beans	**1/4 c**	Balsamic vinegar
3/4 c	Tomatoes, sliced	**2 Tbs**	Fresh lemon juice
1/4 c	Red onion, chopped	**1**	Medium lime
1/2 c	Green bell pepper, chopped		

Preheat grill. Sprinkle the salmon fillets with salt substitute and pepper. Grill for about 6 minutes on each side or until the fish flakes with a fork.

In a mixing bowl, combine the beans, tomatoes, onion, bell pepper, cilantro and jalapeno pepper. In a small mixing bowl, whisk together the garlic, vinegar and lemon juice. Pour over the bean and pepper mixture and toss. Serve fish over the bean salsa. Garnish with lime.

Nutrition Facts

Serving Size 4 oz fillet (292g)
Servings Per Container 4

Amount Per Serving	
Calories 290 Calories from Fat 110	
	% Daily Value
Total Fat 13g	20%
Saturated Fat 3.5g	18%
Trans Fat 0g	
Cholesterol 55mg	18%
Sodium 290mg	12%
Total Carbohydrate 17g	6%
Dietary Fiber 5g	20%
Sugars 4g	
Protein 27g	

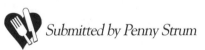 *Submitted by Penny Strum*

SEA BASS PROVENCALE

Number of Servings: 4

1/4 c	Sun dried tomatoes in oil, drained	**1.5 tsp**	Dried thyme
2 Tbs	Extra virgin olive oil	**1/2 c**	White wine
2 Tbs	Capers, drained	**1/2 c**	Clam juice
1 Tbs	Minced garlic	**20 oz**	Sea bass fillets

Preheat oven to 450°. Heat oil in a large skillet over medium-high heat. Add tomatoes, capers, garlic and thyme and stir 1 minute. Add wine and clam juice and boil until liquid is reduced almost to a glaze, about 3 minutes.

Sprinkle fish with pepper. Add to skillet; turn to coat with sauce. Place skillet in oven. Bake fish until just opaque in center, about 15 minutes. Transfer fish and sauce to platter.

Submitted by Jeffrey Wise

Nutrition Facts

Serving Size 5 oz fillet (224g)
Servings Per Container 4

Amount Per Serving

Calories 250 Calories from Fat 100

	% Daily Value
Total Fat 11g	17%
Saturated Fat 2g	10%
Trans Fat 0g	
Cholesterol 60mg	20%
Sodium 310mg	13%
Total Carbohydrate 3g	1%
Dietary Fiber 1g	4%
Sugars 0g	
Protein 27g	

COD PICATTA FLORENTINE

Number of Servings: 4

4	Wild Pacific cod fillets	**2**	Lemons
12 c	Fresh baby spinach	**4 Tbs**	Capers
1 c	Whole wheat flour	**1 Tbs**	Cornstarch
14 oz	Fat free reduced sodium chicken broth	**1 Tbs**	Extra virgin olive oil
		1	Egg white

Sauté the spinach in a large pan with olive oil until just wilted. Pour to make a bed of spinach on a serving platter and keep warm in the oven. Dredge fillets in egg white, then flour (or just the flour) and sauté over medium to medium-high heat in a little olive oil until lightly browned on both sides. DO NOT OVERCOOK THE FISH! Remove and place over warmed spinach and return to oven. Deglaze the sauté pan with juice of 1-1/2 lemons and chicken broth (reserving 1/2 cup to make thickener). Add capers. In a small bowl combine remaining chicken broth and cornstarch; using whisk, mix together to thicken. Add to liquid mixture; heat thoroughly. Pour over the fish and spinach and garnish with lemon slices.

Nutrition Facts

Serving Size 5 oz fillet (433g)
Servings Per Container 4

Amount Per Serving	
Calories 350 Calories from Fat 60	
	% Daily Value
Total Fat 6g	9%
Saturated Fat 1g	5%
Trans Fat 0g	
Cholesterol 45mg	15%
Sodium 650mg	27%
Total Carbohydrate 38g	13%
Dietary Fiber 8g	32%
Sugars 1g	
Protein 37g	

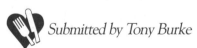

Submitted by Tony Burke

TUNA SALAD

Number of Servings: 4

2 c	White albacore tuna, canned, packed in water, drained and rinsed	**1/4 c**	Plain nonfat yogurt
1/2 c	Celery, diced	**1/4 c**	Light mayonnaise
1/2 c	Green grapes	**1/4 tsp**	Splenda®
		1/8 tsp	Salt substitute
		1/8 c	Slivered almonds
		1/8 c	Walnuts, chopped

Place all ingredients in a large bowl. Stir to mix thoroughly. Chill and serve over fresh green or red leaf lettuce.

Nutrition Facts

Serving Size 1/2 cup (185g)
Servings Per Container 4

Amount Per Serving

Calories 260 Calories from Fat 110

	% Daily Value
Total Fat 13g	20%
Saturated Fat 2g	10%
Trans Fat 0g	
Cholesterol 55mg	18%
Sodium 200mg	8%
Total Carbohydrate 8g	3%
Dietary Fiber 1g	4%
Sugars 5g	
Protein 29g	

When sautéing, use a small amount of chicken broth or wine instead of butter or oil.

FISH ASPARAGUS BAKE

Number of Servings: 3

6	Fresh asparagus, trimmed to 1-inch pieces
3/4 lb	Cod fillets
1/3 c	White onion, chopped
2 Tbs	Trans fat free margarine
1 Tbs	All purpose flour
1/8 tsp	Salt substitute

1 dash	Ground black pepper
3/4 c	Skim milk
1/3 c	2% reduced fat cheddar cheese, shredded
1/4 c	Whole wheat crackers, crushed
1/8 tsp	Parsley flakes

Preheat oven to 350°. In a small saucepan, add asparagus pieces and cover with water. Bring to a boil; cook for 1-2 minutes. Drain and place in a 1-qt. baking dish coated with nonstick cooking spray. Top with fish; set aside.

In a small saucepan, sauté onion in 1 tablespoon margarine until tender. Stir in the flour, salt substitute and pepper until blended. Gradually whisk in milk. Bring to a boil; cook and stir for 1-2 minutes or until thickened. Remove from heat; stir in cheese until melted. Pour over fish.

Melt remaining margarine; stir in crackers and parsley. Sprinkle over cheese sauce. Bake, uncovered, for 20-25 minutes or until crumbs are golden brown and fish flakes easily with a fork.

Nutrition Facts

Serving Size 4 oz fillet (263g)
Servings Per Container 3

Amount Per Serving	
Calories 250	Calories from Fat 80

	% Daily Value
Total Fat 9g	14%
Saturated Fat 2.5g	13%
Trans Fat 0g	
Cholesterol 45mg	15%
Sodium 300mg	13%
Total Carbohydrate 14g	5%
Dietary Fiber 2g	8%
Sugars 5g	
Protein 28g	

VEGGIE QUESADILLAS

Number of Servings: 5

4 oz	Soy cheddar cheese, shredded	**6 oz**	Salsa
1	10-inch whole wheat tortilla	**28 oz**	Fat free sour cream
8 oz	Fat free refried beans	**4**	Fresh jalapeno peppers, sliced

In medium saucepan on low heat add about 1/4 can of water to the refried beans and heat slowly stirring often. When ready, spread a thin layer of the beans over a tortilla and place on a microwave-safe plate. Spread about 2 ounces of soy cheese over the beans and heat on high in the microwave for 20-30 seconds. Spread 2-4 tablespoons of salsa over the cheese and heat thoroughly. Place a second tortilla over the salsa. Heat 20 seconds or more, if necessary to heat throughout. Spread a thin layer of sour cream over the tortilla. Add peppers to taste.

Nutrition Facts

Serving Size 1-10-inch quesadilla (208g)

Servings Per Container 5

Amount Per Serving	
Calories 180 Calories from Fat 30	
	% Daily Value
Total Fat 3.5g	5%
Saturated Fat 0g	0%
Trans Fat 0g	
Cholesterol 5mg	2%
Sodium 750mg	31%
Total Carbohydrate 23g	8%
Dietary Fiber 4g	16%
Sugars 2g	
Protein 11g	

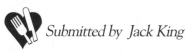 *Submitted by Jack King*

FAUX PIMENTO CHEESE SPREAD

Number of Servings: 4

7 oz	Soy cheddar cheese, shredded	**2 Tbs**	Fat free mayonnaise
3-1/2 oz	Sliced pimentos, drained & rinsed	**1/4 Tbs**	Ground black pepper
		1/4 Tbs	Original blend Mrs. Dash®

In a mixing bowl, combine soy cheese shreds and the sliced pimentos. Add fat free mayonnaise, pepper and salt substitute. Break long shreds of cheese with a fork. Mix well. Refrigerate until ready to serve. Enjoy with whole wheat crackers or as a grilled cheese sandwich.

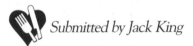 *Submitted by Jack King*

Nutrition Facts

Serving Size 2 tablespoons (83g)
Servings Per Container 4

Amount Per Serving

Calories 120   Calories from Fat 50

	% Daily Value
Total Fat 6g	9%
Saturated Fat 0g	0%
Trans Fat 0g	
Cholesterol 0mg	0%
Sodium 650mg	27%
Total Carbohydrate 2g	1%
Dietary Fiber 1g	4%
Sugars 1g	
Protein 13g	

Bean Math
- One 15-ounce can of beans = 1 1/2 cups cooked beans, drained.
- One pound dry beans = six cups cooked beans, drained.
- One pound dry beans = two cups dry beans.
- One cup dry beans = three cups cooked beans, drained.

CHICKEN SALAD SPREAD

Number of Servings: 12

2 lbs	Boneless skinless chicken breasts, cooked	**2 Tbs**	Sweet pickle relish
1/3 c	Celery, diced	**1/4 c**	Fat free mayonnaise
1/4 c	Vidalia onion, chopped	**1/4 c**	Light mayonnaise
2	Omega-3 eggs, hard boiled, chopped	**1/8 tsp**	Paprika
		1 dash	Ground black pepper

Place the cooked chicken into a food processor and process until finely ground. Add remaining ingredients and blend well. Refrigerate for at least one hour. Spread on your favorite whole wheat cracker, whole wheat pita or whole wheat bread.

Nutrition Facts

Serving Size 1/4 cup (101g)
Servings Per Container 12

Amount Per Serving

Calories 120   Calories from Fat 40

	% Daily Value
Total Fat 4g	6%
Saturated Fat 0g	0%
Trans Fat 0g	
Cholesterol 65mg	22%
Sodium 480mg	20%
Total Carbohydrate 3g	1%
Dietary Fiber 0g	0%
Sugars 1g	
Protein 19g	

PEPPER PITAS

Number of Servings: 2

1/2 c	Fat free cream cheese	**3 oz**	Yellow bell peppers, sliced
2 Tbs	Salsa	**4 oz**	White onion, chopped
1	Whole wheat pita bread	**2 tsp**	Extra virgin olive oil
3 oz	Red bell peppers, sliced	**1/2 tsp**	Hot pepper sauce
3 oz	Green bell peppers, sliced	**1/8 tsp**	Ground black pepper

In a small mixing bowl, beat cream cheese until smooth. Beat in salsa. Spread cream cheese mixture inside pita halves; set aside. In a nonstick skillet, sauté peppers and onion in oil until tender. Add hot pepper sauce, pepper and salt substitute. Spoon about 1/4 cup into each pita half.

Nutrition Facts

Serving Size 1 filled pita half (284g)
Servings Per Container 2

Amount Per Serving	
Calories 220	Calories from Fat 60

	% Daily Value
Total Fat 6g	9%
Saturated Fat 1.5g	8%
Trans Fat 0g	
Cholesterol 5mg	2%
Sodium 530mg	22%
Total Carbohydrate 30g	10%
Dietary Fiber 4g	16%
Sugars 7g	
Protein 12g	

If you experience chest pain for the first time and it lasts longer than 10 minutes, call your doctor. If you can't reach your doctor promptly, call 911.

BISTRO CHICKEN

Number of Servings: 4

2 tsp	Canola oil	**1 lb**	Boneless skinless chicken breasts
3 c	Mushrooms, sliced		
1/2 c	White onion, chopped	**1/3 c**	Reduced fat mozzarella cheese, shredded
1	15 oz can no salt added diced tomatoes		
1/4 c	Fat free Italian salad dressing	**2 Tbs**	Turkey bacon, cooked, crumbled
3 Tbs	No salt added tomato paste		

Heat oil in a large nonstick skillet on medium-high heat. Add mushrooms and onions; cook 5 minutes, stirring occasionally. Stir in tomatoes with their liquid, the dressing and tomato paste. Add chicken; cover. Reduce heat to medium-low. Simmer 12 minutes or until chicken is cooked through. Sprinkle with cheese and bacon; simmer, uncovered, 5 minutes or until cheese is melted. Serve over brown rice, if desired.

Nutrition Facts

Serving Size 3 oz breast (335g)
Servings Per Container 4

Amount Per Serving

Calories 240   Calories from Fat 60

	% Daily Value
Total Fat 6g	9%
Saturated Fat 1.5g	8%
Trans Fat 0g	
Cholesterol 75mg	25%
Sodium 470mg	20%
Total Carbohydrate 12g	4%
Dietary Fiber 2g	8%
Sugars 7g	
Protein 33g	

CHICKEN PICCATA

Number of Servings: 4

12 oz	Boneless skinless chicken breasts
2 Tbs	All purpose flour
1/2 tsp	Paprika
1 tsp	Ground black pepper
1 Tbs	Trans fat free margarine
1-1/2 Tbs	Extra virgin olive oil
1/4 c	Sweet Marsala dessert wine
1/4 c	Fresh lemon juice
2 Tbs	Fresh lemon rind, grated
2 Tbs	Capers, canned, drained

Placing each breast between plastic wrap, pound out to 1/4-inch thickness (can be thinner but not paper thin). Combine flour, paprika and pepper in a shallow dish. Dust each breast with flour mixture. In a large skillet, melt margarine and olive oil over medium-high heat. If skillet is not big enough to fit all four breasts, work in batches, browning each breast 2 minutes per side. Remove from pan and keep warm.

Deglaze the pan with the wine, scraping all the brown bits from the bottom. Add the lemon juice and grated lemon rind and return chicken to the pan. Add the capers and cook for an additional 2 minutes making sure everything is warm. Serve with brown rice or favorite vegetable and pour any left over sauce over chicken.

Nutrition Facts

Serving Size 1 chicken breast (136g)
Servings Per Container 4

Amount Per Serving

Calories 210   Calories from Fat 80

	% Daily Value
Total Fat 9g	14%
Saturated Fat 1.5g	8%
Trans Fat 0g	
Cholesterol 50mg	17%
Sodium 350mg	15%
Total Carbohydrate 7g	2%
Dietary Fiber 1g	4%
Sugars 2g	
Protein 21g	

GREEK CHICKEN AND RICE SKILLET

Number of Servings: 6

1/3 c	Green Goddess salad dressing	**1-1/4 c**	Green bell peppers, chopped
1 lb	Boneless skinless chicken breasts, diced	**1-1/4 c**	Carrots, chopped
2 tsp	Dried oregano leaves, whole	**15 oz**	Fat free reduced sodium chicken broth
1-1/4 c	Broccoli florets, chopped	**2 c**	Instant brown rice
		1	Lemon

Heat dressing in a large deep nonstick skillet on medium heat. Add chicken; sprinkle with oregano. Cook 5 minutes, stirring once. Add vegetables and broth; simmer 5 minutes. Stir in rice; cover. Simmer 5 minutes. Turn off heat. Let stand, covered, 5 minutes or until liquid is absorbed. Grate 1 teaspoon lemon peel; sprinkle over chicken. Cut lemon into 4 wedges; serve with chicken and rice mixture, if desired.

Nutrition Facts

Serving Size 1 cup (275g)
Servings Per Container 6

Amount Per Serving	
Calories 270	Calories from Fat 60

	% Daily Value
Total Fat 7g	11%
Saturated Fat 1g	5%
Trans Fat 0g	
Cholesterol 45mg	15%
Sodium 390mg	16%
Total Carbohydrate 30g	10%
Dietary Fiber 3g	12%
Sugars 2g	
Protein 22g	

If you stick with something for 21 days, it will become a habit. Keep a journal for 21 days or mark it on a calendar. Before you know it, your healthy habits will be your lifestyle.

PARMESAN CHICKEN WITH CREAM SAUCE

Number of Servings: 4

2 c	Brown rice	**1 lb**	Boneless skinless chicken breasts
14 oz	Fat free reduced sodium chicken broth	**2 tsp**	Canola oil
1/4 c	Whole wheat crackers, crushed	**1/3 c**	Roasted garlic flavored light cream cheese
2 Tbs	Parmesan cheese, grated	**3/4 lb**	Cooked asparagus spears

Cook rice as directed on package, using 1-1/4 cups of the broth and 1/2 cup water.

Meanwhile, mix cracker crumbs and parmesan cheese on plate. Rinse chicken breasts with cold water; shake off excess water. Dip chicken in cracker mixture, turning to coat.

Nutrition Facts

Serving Size 3 oz breast (641g)
Servings Per Container 4

Amount Per Serving

Calories 610 Calories from Fat 100

	% Daily Value
Total Fat 12g	18%
Saturated Fat 4g	20%
Trans Fat 0g	
Cholesterol 80mg	27%
Sodium 500mg	21%
Total Carbohydrate 84g	28%
Dietary Fiber 8g	32%
Sugars 2g	
Protein 39g	

Heat oil in large nonstick skillet on medium heat. Add chicken; cook 5-6 minutes on each side or until chicken is cooked through. Place chicken on serving plate. Set aside; keep warm. Add remaining 1/2 cup broth and cream cheese spread to same skillet. Cook on medium heat until mixture just comes to a boil, stirring constantly. Simmer 3 minutes or until sauce thickens. Spoon sauce over chicken. Serve rice and asparagus with chicken.

TASTY TURKEY BURGERS

Number of Servings: 4

1/4 c	Green bell pepper, chopped	**1/4 c**	Fresh parsley, chopped
1/2 c	White onion, chopped	**1/2 c**	Fat free parmesan cheese
3 Tbs	No salt added tomato paste	**1 tsp**	Salt substitute
2	Garlic cloves	**1 Tbs**	Extra virgin olive oil
1 Tbs	Worcestershire sauce	**1 lb**	99% fat free ground turkey

Combine meat with all the ingredients, except olive oil. Form turkey into 4 large patties or 5 medium ones. Drizzle extra virgin olive oil on patties and cook for 5-6 minutes on each side in a hot skillet. Remove burgers from skillet and drain on a paper towel. Serve with a whole wheat bun.

Nutrition Facts

Serving Size 3 oz cooked (61g)
Servings Per Container 4

Amount Per Serving	
Calories 70	Calories from Fat 15

	% Daily Value
Total Fat 1.5g	2%
Saturated Fat 0g	0%
Trans Fat 0g	
Cholesterol 15mg	5%
Sodium 105mg	4%
Total Carbohydrate 2g	1%
Dietary Fiber 0g	0%
Sugars 1g	
Protein 11g	

For low-salt grilling, try a combination of lime juice and chili powder as a salt substitute.

PEACHY PORK TENDERLOIN

Number of Servings: 8

1/4 c	Splenda®	**2 Tbs**	Low sodium
1/4 c	Brown sugar, packed		soy sauce
2 Tbs	Cornstarch	**1**	15 oz can peaches
1 Tbs	Mustard		in own syrup, diced
2/3 c	Apple cider vinegar	**2 lb**	Lean pork tenderloin
1/2 c	Water		

Preheat oven to 350°. In a heavy saucepan, combine the first 8 ingredients over moderate heat and stir until slightly thickened. Brown the pork tenderloins in a skillet sprayed with nonstick cooking spray over medium to medium-high heat. Place browned tenderloins in a 9x13-inch pan and pour sauce over the top. Bake uncovered, for 1-1/4 hours adding water, if needed, to keep from drying out. Cut cooked tenderloins into medallions, place on platter and pour sauce from pan over meat before serving.

Nutrition Facts

Serving Size 3-1-inch medallions (216g)

Servings Per Container 8

Amount Per Serving

Calories 210   Calories from Fat 35

	% Daily Value
Total Fat 4g	6%
Saturated Fat 1.5g	8%
Trans Fat 0g	
Cholesterol 75mg	25%
Sodium 220mg	9%
Total Carbohydrate 18g	6%
Dietary Fiber 1g	4%
Sugars 12g	
Protein 24g	

Not all fat is created equal. Fat around the middle of your body is more dangerous than fat on your hips and thighs.

BEEF ENCHILADAS

Number of Servings: 8

8	6-inch whole wheat tortillas	**1 c**	Chunky salsa
1/2 lb	96% lean ground beef	**1/2 c**	2% reduced fat cheddar cheese, shredded
1/2 c	Green bell peppers, chopped		
1/2 c	Red bell peppers, chopped	**2 Tbs**	Fresh cilantro, chopped

Preheat oven to 400°. Cook meat and peppers in large nonstick skillet on medium heat until meat is no longer pink, stirring frequently. Add 1 cup of the salsa; simmer 3-4 minutes or until peppers are tender. Remove from heat; stir in 1/2 cup of the cheese.

Spread 1/4 cup of the salsa on bottom of 13x9-inch baking dish. Stack 4 of the tortillas and wrap them in a large sheet of waxed paper. Microwave on HIGH 20-30 seconds or just until warm. Immediately spoon 1/3 cup meat mixture down center of each warm tortilla; roll up. Place, seam side down, in dish. Repeat with remaining 4 tortillas and remaining meat mixture. Spoon remaining 3/4 cup salsa evenly over filled tortillas; cover with foil.

Bake 20 minutes or until heated through. Uncover; top with remaining 1/2 cup cheese. Bake an additional 2-3 minutes or until cheese is melted. Top with chopped cilantro.

Nutrition Facts

Serving Size 1 enchilada (122g)
Servings Per Container 8

Amount Per Serving

Calories 140   Calories from Fat 30

	% Daily Value
Total Fat 3g	5%
Saturated Fat 1.5g	8%
Trans Fat 0g	
Cholesterol 20mg	7%
Sodium 460mg	19%
Total Carbohydrate 23g	8%
Dietary Fiber 3g	12%
Sugars 2g	
Protein 10g	

BROCCOLI COLESLAW

Number of Servings: 8

1	Red onion	**2 Tbs**	Splenda®
1/4 c	Light mayonnaise	**1 tsp**	Celery seeds
1/4 c	Plain nonfat yogurt	**1/2 tsp**	Paprika
1/4 c	Fat free sour cream	**4 c**	Broccoli slaw
1/4 c	Reduced fat parmesan cheese, grated	**5 c**	Cabbage slaw

In a large salad bowl combine the cabbage and broccoli slaws and onion. In a small mixing bowl, combine the remaining ingredients. Toss to coat and refrigerate until ready to serve.

Nutrition Facts

Serving Size 1/2 cup (75g)
Servings Per Container 8

Amount Per Serving

Calories 40   Calories from Fat 15

	% Daily Value
Total Fat 1.5g	2%
Saturated Fat 0g	0%
Trans Fat 0g	
Cholesterol 5mg	2%
Sodium 80mg	3%
Total Carbohydrate 6g	2%
Dietary Fiber 2g	8%
Sugars 2g	
Protein 2g	

CREAMY POTATO SALAD

Number of Servings: 16

2 lb	Red potatoes, with skin		**1 c**	Fat free sour cream
1-1/2 c	Celery, diced		**4 tsp**	Mustard
1/2 c	Red onion, chopped		**1/2 tsp**	Salt substitute
4 Tbs	Pickle relish		**1 tsp**	Celery seeds
1/2 c	Light mayonnaise		**2**	Omega-3 eggs, hardboiled, chopped
1/2 c	Fat free mayonnaise			

In a large covered saucepan, cook the potatoes in boiling water for 20-25 minutes or until just tender. Drain well and cool slightly. Peel and cube the potatoes. Transfer to a large bowl. Add celery, onion and pickle relish. In a small bowl, mix together the mayonnaise, sour cream, milk, mustard, salt substitute and celery seed. Pour over potatoes. Toss lightly to coat potatoes and add egg. Cover and refrigerate for at least 4 or up to 24 hours before serving.

Nutrition Facts

Serving Size 1/4 cup (116g)
Servings Per Container 16

Amount Per Serving

Calories 100   Calories from Fat 30

	% Daily Value
Total Fat 3.5g	5%
Saturated Fat 0g	0%
Trans Fat 0g	
Cholesterol 25mg	8%
Sodium 180mg	8%
Total Carbohydrate 15g	5%
Dietary Fiber 1g	4%
Sugars 3g	
Protein 3g	

BROWN RICE WITH LEMON AND SHALLOTS

Number of Servings: 12

1 Tbs	Extra virgin olive oil	**1/2 tsp**	Sugar
1/2 c	Shallots, chopped	**1/2 tsp**	Ground black pepper
2 tsp	Minced garlic	**1-1/2 c**	Fat free reduced
1 Tbs	Lemon juice		sodium chicken broth
1 Tbs	Fresh parsley, chopped	**3/4 c**	Brown rice, cooked

Warm oil in a medium size saucepan over medium heat. Add the shallots and garlic. Sauté for 3 minutes. Add the lemon juice, parsley, sugar and pepper. Stir in the broth and bring to a boil. Add the rice and reduce heat to medium-low. Cover and simmer for 35-40 minutes or until the broth is absorbed. Remove rice from heat. Fluff lightly with a fork and keep covered until serving time.

Nutrition Facts

Serving Size 1/2 cup (76g)
Servings Per Container 12

Amount Per Serving

Calories 60   Calories from Fat 15

	% Daily Value
Total Fat 1.5g	2%
Saturated Fat 0g	0%
Trans Fat 0g	
Cholesterol 0mg	0%
Sodium 60mg	3%
Total Carbohydrate 11g	4%
Dietary Fiber 1g	4%
Sugars 0g	
Protein 1g	

WHOLEGRAIN MUFFINS

Number of Servings: 12

3/4 c	1% milk	**1/8 c**	Brown sugar, packed
3/4 c	Wheat bran	**1 c**	Old fashioned oats
2	Egg whites	**2/3 c**	Whole wheat flour
1/4 c	Canola oil	**1 Tbs**	Baking powder
1/8 c	Honey	**1/2 c**	Walnuts, chopped

Preheat oven to 400°. Combine milk and wheat bran in medium sized bowl. Add egg whites, oil, honey, brown sugar; mix well. Add remaining ingredients, mixing just until dry ingredients are moistened. Fill 12 greased or paper-lined medium sized muffin cups 2/3 full. Bake 15 minutes.

Nutrition Facts

Serving Size 1 muffin (55g)
Servings Per Container 12

Amount Per Serving	
Calories 160	Calories from Fat 80

	% Daily Value
Total Fat 9g	14%
Saturated Fat 1g	5%
Trans Fat 0g	
Cholesterol 0mg	0%
Sodium 120mg	5%
Total Carbohydrate 18g	6%
Dietary Fiber 3g	12%
Sugars 6g	
Protein 4g	

Legumes may cause intestinal discomfort. You can minimize this effect by changing the soaking water several times when you prepare dried beans, or switching to canned beans. When canned, some of the gas-producing substances are eliminated. Be sure to rinse the beans well to wash off excess salt. Another option is "Beano," which contains an enzyme that breaks down gas-producing substances in the beans. CDC.gov – 5 a Day

MIXED BERRY SMOOTHIE

Number of Servings: 4

2 c	Skim milk	**1 c**	Frozen mixed fruit
6 oz	Lowfat strawberry yogurt	**2**	Large shredded wheat cereal biscuits, crumbled
1	Small box of sugar free strawberry gelatin		

Combine all ingredients in a blender. Cover. Blend on high for 15 seconds or until smooth.

Nutrition Facts

Serving Size 1 cup (214g)
Servings Per Container 4

Amount Per Serving

Calories 150   Calories from Fat 5

	% Daily Value
Total Fat 0.5g	1%
Saturated Fat 0g	0%
Trans Fat 0g	
Cholesterol 5mg	2%
Sodium 100mg	4%
Total Carbohydrate 28g	9%
Dietary Fiber 3g	12%
Sugars 15g	
Protein 8g	

EASY JELLO® DESSERT

Number of Servings: 4

1	Small box of sugar free strawberry gelatin	**1/2 c**	Cold water
3/4 c	Boiling water	**1/2 c**	Fat free whipped topping

Dissolve dry gelatin mix in 3/4 cup boiling water. Add enough ice cubes to 1/2 cup cold water to measure 1-1/4 cups; add to gelatin mixture. Pour into blender; cover and blend 30 seconds. Add whipping topping; cover and blend until smooth. Pour evenly into 4 dessert dishes. Refrigerate at least 20 minutes or until set. Store left over dessert in refrigerator.

Nutrition Facts

Serving Size 1/2 cup (84g)
Servings Per Container 4

Amount Per Serving

Calories 15   Calories from Fat 0

	% Daily Value
Total Fat 0g	0%
Saturated Fat 0g	0%
Trans Fat 0g	
Cholesterol 0mg	0%
Sodium 20mg	1%
Total Carbohydrate 3g	1%
Dietary Fiber 0g	0%
Sugars 1g	
Protein 0g	

STRAWBERRY FRUIT PIE.

Number of Servings: 8

1-1/2 c Water
1 Small box of sugar
  free strawberry gelatin

2 pt Strawberries, sliced
4 squares Low fat graham
  crackers, crushed

Spray a 9-inch pie plate with nonstick cooking spray. In a large bowl, stir together boiling water and gelatin for 2 minutes or until dissolved. Add 1 cup ice cubes, stirring until melted. Refrigerate 30 minutes or until slightly thickened. Stir in strawberries. Pour into pie plate. Sprinkle graham cracker crumbs around edge of pie. Refrigerate 3 hours or until firm.

Nutrition Facts

Serving Size 2-inch wedge (129g)
Servings Per Container 8

Amount Per Serving

Calories 35	Calories from Fat 5

	% Daily Value
Total Fat 0g	0%
Saturated Fat 0g	0%
Trans Fat 0g	
Cholesterol 0mg	0%
Sodium 15mg	1%
Total Carbohydrate 8g	3%
Dietary Fiber 2g	8%
Sugars 4g	
Protein 1g	

PINEAPPLE AND CHEESE CASSEROLE

Number of Servings: 8

2 lb	Canned pineapple chunks, not drained	**1 c**	Splenda®
6 oz	2% reduced fat sharp cheddar cheese, shredded	**6**	Low fat graham crackers
2 Tbs	All purpose flour	**3 Tbs**	Trans fat free margarine

Preheat oven to 350°. Drain pineapple; reserve juice. In a large bowl mix pineapple chunks, cheese, flour, Splenda® and pineapple juice. Pour pineapple mixture into 2 quart casserole dish coated with cooking spray. Sprinkle crushed graham cracker crumbs over mixture and top with margarine. Bake for 45 minutes.

Nutrition Facts

Serving Size 1/2 cup (150g)
Servings Per Container 8

Amount Per Serving

Calories 170   Calories from Fat 70

	% Daily Value
Total Fat 8g	12%
Saturated Fat 3.5g	18%
Trans Fat 0g	
Cholesterol 15mg	5%
Sodium 230mg	10%
Total Carbohydrate 19g	6%
Dietary Fiber 1g	4%
Sugars 10g	
Protein 6g	

PINEAPPLE ANGEL LUSH

Number of Servings: 10

2	Small boxes of sugar free vanilla pudding	**1 c**	Fat free whipped topping
20 oz	Canned crushed pineapple in light syrup	**1**	Sugar free angel food cake
		10	Medium strawberries, sliced

Mix dry pudding mix and pineapple with juice in medium bowl. Gently stir in whipped topping. Cut cake horizontally into 3 layers. Place bottom cake layer, cut side up, on serving plate. Spread 1-1/3 cups of the pudding mixture onto cake layer; cover with middle cake layer. Spread 1 cup of the pudding mixture onto middle cake layer; top with remaining cake layer. Spread with remaining pudding mixture. Refrigerate at least 1 hour or until ready to serve. Garnish with sliced strawberries. Store in refrigerator.

Nutrition Facts

Serving Size 2-inch wedge (118g)
Servings Per Container 10

Amount Per Serving	
Calories 130	Calories from Fat 0

	% Daily Value
Total Fat 0g	0%
Saturated Fat 0g	0%
Trans Fat 0g	
Cholesterol 0mg	0%
Sodium 310mg	13%
Total Carbohydrate 29g	10%
Dietary Fiber 1g	4%
Sugars 9g	
Protein 2g	

CHOCOLATE PUDDING PIE

Number of Servings: 8

2 c Soy milk
1 c Fat free
whipped topping
1 Small box of sugar free
instant chocolate
pudding mix

1 9-inch reduced fat
graham cracker crust

Make pudding with the 2 cups of soy milk. Pour into crust. Refrigerate 1-2 hours until firm. Spread 1 cup of fat free whipped topping over the top of the pie. Keep refrigerated.

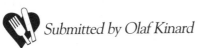 *Submitted by Olaf Kinard*

Nutrition Facts

Serving Size 1/8 slice (74g)
Servings Per Container 8

Amount Per Serving	
Calories 50	Calories from Fat 10

	% Daily Value
Total Fat 1.5g	2%
Saturated Fat 0g	0%
Trans Fat 0g	
Cholesterol 0mg	0%
Sodium 80mg	3%
Total Carbohydrate 7g	2%
Dietary Fiber 1g	4%
Sugars 1g	
Protein 3g	

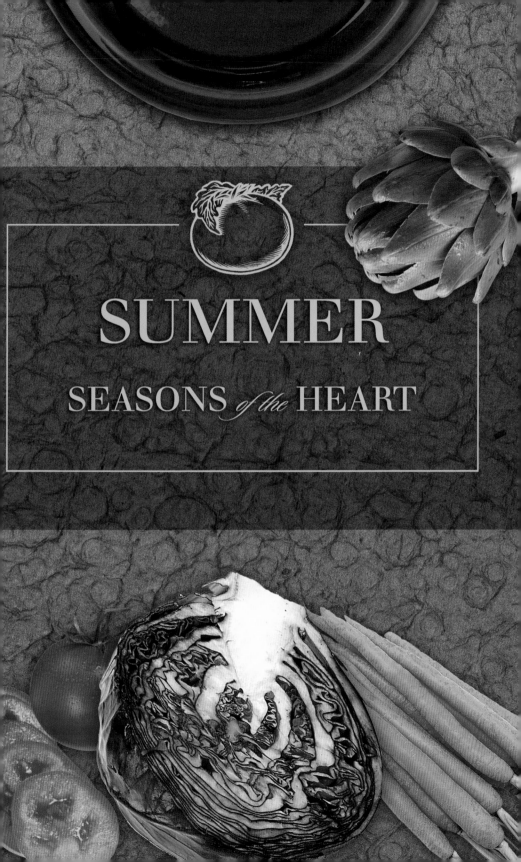

SUMMER

SEASONS *of the* HEART

RASPBERRY SWEET TEA

Number of Servings: 15

4 qt   Water
1 c   Splenda®
10   Small decaf tea bags

12 oz   Frozen raspberries, thawed & not drained
3 Tbs   Fresh lime juice

In a large saucepan, bring 2 of the 4 quarts of water to a boil. Stir in Splenda® until dissolved. Remove from heat. Add tea bags; steep for 5-8 minutes. Discard tea bags.

In another saucepan, bring raspberries and remaining water to a boil. Reduce heat; simmer, uncovered, for 3 minutes. Strain and discard pulp. Add raspberry juice and lime juice to the tea. Transfer to a large pitcher. Refrigerate until chilled.

Nutrition Facts

Serving Size 1 cup (281g)
Servings Per Container 15

Amount Per Serving	
Calories 15	Calories from Fat 0
	% Daily Value
Total Fat 0g	0%
Saturated Fat 0g	0%
Trans Fat 0g	
Cholesterol 0mg	0%
Sodium 5mg	0%
Total Carbohydrate 4g	1%
Dietary Fiber 0g	0%
Sugars 1g	
Protein 0g	

Make your own white sauce using 2 tablespoons reduced-fat margarine, 2 tablespoons flour and 1 cup skim milk. Add fat free cheese slices for a great cheese sauce.

NICOLE'S TEXAS CAVIAR

Number of Servings: 16

1	11 oz can 50% less salt corn	**1 c**	Tomatoes, chopped
1	15 oz can 50% less salt black beans	**3/4 c**	Green bell pepper, chopped
1	15 oz can fat free no salt added kidney beans	**3/4 c**	Red onion, chopped
1	15 oz can black eyed peas	**16 oz**	Fat free Italian salad dressing

Drain and rinse all canned products. Combine all ingredients in a large bowl and mix well. Cover and refrigerate. Serve with natural tortilla chips, if desired.

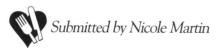 *Submitted by Nicole Martin*

Nutrition Facts

Serving Size 1/2 cup (155g)
Servings Per Container 16

Amount Per Serving

Calories 100	Calories from Fat 5
	% Daily Value
Total Fat 0g	0%
Saturated Fat 0g	0%
Trans Fat 0g	
Cholesterol 0mg	0%
Sodium 250mg	12%
Total Carbohydrate 19g	6%
Dietary Fiber 5g	20%
Sugars 4g	
Protein 5g	

GAZPACHO

Number of Servings: 4

4	Tomatoes, chopped	**3**	Garlic cloves, chopped
1	Cucumber, chopped	**1/4 c**	Hot pepper sauce
1/3 c	Red bell pepper, chopped	**1/4 c**	Red wine vinegar
1/3 c	Green bell pepper, chopped	**3 Tbs**	Extra virgin olive oil
1/3 oz	Red onion, chopped	**2 Tbs**	Fresh basil, chopped
		2 c	Frozen no salt added mixed vegetables

Place chopped vegetables into food processor or blender. Add hot sauce, vinegar, oil and basil. Process until smooth. Transfer soup to large glass serving bowl. Thaw and drain mixed vegetables. Stir in additional mixed vegetables. Cover and refrigerate one hour before serving.

Nutrition Facts

Serving Size 1 cup (418g)
Servings Per Container 4

Amount Per Serving	
Calories 210 Calories from Fat 100	
	% Daily Value
Total Fat 11g	17%
Saturated Fat 1.5g	8%
Trans Fat 0g	
Cholesterol 0mg	0%
Sodium 420mg	18%
Total Carbohydrate 24g	8%
Dietary Fiber 7g	28%
Sugars 10g	
Protein 5g	

TOMATO BASIL SALAD

Number of Servings: 4

4	Tomatoes, 1/2" thick slices	**1/2 c**	Light mozzarella cheese, shredded
1	Red onion, thinly sliced	**1/3 c**	Balsamic vinegar salad dressing
1/2 c	Fresh basil, chopped		

Arrange tomatoes, onion and basil on serving platter; sprinkle with cheese. Drizzle with dressing. Serve immediately.

Nutrition Facts

Serving Size 1 tomato and 2-3 slices onion(72g)
Servings Per Container 4

Amount Per Serving

Calories 70   Calories from Fat 20

	% Daily Value
Total Fat 2g	3%
Saturated Fat 1.5g	8%
Trans Fat 0g	
Cholesterol 10mg	3%
Sodium 410mg	17%
Total Carbohydrate 7g	2%
Dietary Fiber 1g	4%
Sugars 6g	
Protein 4g	

Heart disease is the #1 killer of women over the age of 50.

EGG SALAD

Number of Servings: 12

6	Hard boiled omega-3 eggs	**1/2 tsp**	Celery seeds
4 Tbs	Light mayonnaise	**1 Dash**	Ground black pepper
2 Tbs	Sweet pickle relish	**1 c**	Romaine lettuce, chopped
2 tsp	Dijon mustard		

Chop and combine 3 egg yolks and all 6 egg whites. Discard the remaining 3 yolks. Add remaining ingredients; mix well. Refrigerate at least one hour. Serve over lettuce. Garnish with cherry tomatoes if desired.

Nutrition Facts

Serving Size 1/4 cup (51g)
Servings Per Container 12

Amount Per Serving

Calories 80   Calories from Fat 50

	% Daily Value
Total Fat 5g	8%
Saturated Fat 1.5g	8%
Trans Fat 0g	
Cholesterol 145mg	48%
Sodium 120mg	5%
Total Carbohydrate 2g	1%
Dietary Fiber 0g	0%
Sugars 1g	
Protein 5g	

CANDY'S QUICK AND EASY PASTA SALAD

Number of Servings: 8

16 oz Whole wheat rotini pasta
10 oz Frozen cut green beans
10 oz Frozen green bell peppers, chopped

1/2 c Light zesty Italian salad dressing, bottled
8 oz Chicken breast strips, grilled

In a medium saucepan, cook pasta as directed on package. Cut chicken breasts into pieces. Right before the pasta is to be drained, add bean and pepper mix. Allow frozen vegetables to heat through, then drain pasta, beans and peppers. Add dressing to coat pasta and vegetables. Serve hot or cold.

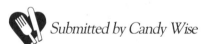 *Submitted by Candy Wise*

Nutrition Facts

Serving Size 1/2 cup (171g)
Servings Per Container 8

Amount Per Serving	
Calories 160	Calories from Fat 20

	% Daily Value
Total Fat 2g	3%
Saturated Fat 0g	0%
Trans Fat 0g	
Cholesterol 15mg	5%
Sodium 250mg	10%
Total Carbohydrate 23g	8%
Dietary Fiber 2g	8%
Sugars 1g	
Protein 11g	

PIMENTO CHEESE SPREAD

Number of Servings: 16

2 c	Fat free cheddar cheese, shredded	**1/2 tsp**	Hot pepper sauce
1 c	Fat free mozzarella cheese, shredded	**1/2 c**	Low sodium Worcestershire sauce
1/2 c	Light mayonnaise	**2 oz**	Sliced pimentos
1/2 c	Fat free mayonnaise	**1**	14 oz can no salt added tomatoes

In a large mixing bowl combine the cheese and mayonnaise first, then add remaining ingredients. Refrigerate for at least one hour before serving.

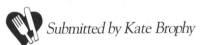 *Submitted by Kate Brophy*

Nutrition Facts

Serving Size 2 tablespoons (67g)
Servings Per Container 16

Amount Per Serving

Calories 70   Calories from Fat 25

	% Daily Value
Total Fat 2.5g	4%
Saturated Fat 0g	0%
Trans Fat 0g	
Cholesterol 5mg	2%
Sodium 280mg	12%
Total Carbohydrate 4g	1%
Dietary Fiber 0g	0%
Sugars 2g	
Protein 7g	

GROUPER KEY LARGO

Number of Servings: 2

10 oz	Grouper fillets	**2 tsp**	Cornstarch
4 tsp	Dijon mustard	**4 tsp**	Fresh parsley,
1 c	Skim milk		chopped
2 tsp	Lime juice		

To prepare sauce, combine mustard, skim milk and lime juice in a saucepan. Bring to a simmer. Add cornstarch, stir continuously and simmer until desired consistency. Grill grouper over medium-hot grill until fish flakes with a fork. Remove from grill and place on serving plate. Pour sauce over fish and sprinkle with chopped parsley. Note: The grouper may also be baked or broiled in the oven.

Nutrition Facts

Serving Size 5 oz fillet (287g)
Servings Per Container 2

Amount Per Serving

Calories 200   Calories from Fat 20

% Daily Value

Total Fat 2.5g	4%
Saturated Fat 0g	0%
Trans Fat 0g	
Cholesterol 55mg	18%
Sodium 390mg	16%
Total Carbohydrate 11g	4%
Dietary Fiber 0g	0%
Sugars 6g	
Protein 33g	

Use de-fatted broth, fruit juice, wine, water or cider to sauté meats and vegetables instead of oil or butter.

CITRUS MARINATED MONKFISH

Number of Servings: 4

1 lb	Monkfish	**2 Tbs**	Fresh basil leaves, chopped
1/4 c	Orange juice	**1/4 tsp**	Salt substitute
2 Tbs	Lemon juice	**1/4 tsp**	Ground black pepper
2 Tbs	Lime juice		
2 Tbs	Canola oil		

Preheat grill to medium-high heat. In a large bowl, whisk together orange juice, lemon juice, lime juice, oil, basil, salt substitute and pepper. Add monkfish to bowl and marinate for at least 30 minutes. Grill fish, covered with grill lid, over medium-high heat for 5-7 minutes or until fish is opaque.

Nutrition Facts

Serving Size 4 oz fillet (153g)
Servings Per Container 4

Amount Per Serving

Calories 160   Calories from Fat 80

	% Daily Value
Total Fat 9g	14%
Saturated Fat 1g	5%
Trans Fat 0g	
Cholesterol 30mg	10%
Sodium 20mg	1%
Total Carbohydrate 3g	1%
Dietary Fiber 0g	0%
Sugars 2g	
Protein 17g	

MAHI MAHI WITH CILANTRO AND LIME

Number of Servings: 4

2	Shallots, chopped	**1/4 tsp**	Salt substitute
1/4 c	Cilantro	**1/4 tsp**	Ground black pepper
1/2 c	Lime juice	**1 lb**	Mahi Mahi fillets
2 Tbs	Extra virgin olive oil		

Preheat grill and coat rack with nonstick cooking spray. Combine shallots, cilantro, lime juice, olive oil, salt and pepper in a medium bowl. Pour over Mahi Mahi. Grill covered, over medium-high heat 6-8 minutes or until fish flakes with a fork.

Nutrition Facts

Serving Size 4 oz fillet (158g)
Servings Per Container 4

Amount Per Serving	
Calories 170 Calories from Fat 70	
	% Daily Value
Total Fat 8g	12%
Saturated Fat 1g	5%
Trans Fat 0g	
Cholesterol 85mg	28%
Sodium 100mg	4%
Total Carbohydrate 4g	1%
Dietary Fiber 0g	0%
Sugars 1g	
Protein 21g	

ORANGE ROUGHY PRIMAVERA

Number of Servings: 4

1/2	Zucchini squash, sliced thick	**1/2**	Carrot, sliced thick
1/2	Red bell pepper, sliced thick	**1 tsp**	Fresh rosemary
		1 tsp	Thyme
1/2	Yellow onion, sliced thick	**1 tsp**	Ground black pepper
		2 Tbs	Extra virgin olive oil
		20 oz	Orange Roughy fillets

Preheat grill. In a large bowl, combine the rosemary, thyme, pepper and oil; add vegetables and coat with one half of the herb oil. Place the vegetables on the grill; close and cook until tender.

Remove the vegetables and add the fillets. Drizzle the remaining herb oil over the fillets and close the grill. If needed, place foil on grill, spray with nonstick cooking spray and place fish on foil. Cook for 2-3 minutes on each side. Continue grilling fish until it flakes easily. To serve, carefully remove the fillets from the grill and top with the vegetables.

Nutrition Facts

Serving Size 5 oz fillet (194g)
Servings Per Container 4

Amount Per Serving

Calories 180   Calories from Fat 70

	% Daily Value
Total Fat 8g	12%
Saturated Fat 1g	5%
Trans Fat 0g	
Cholesterol 30mg	10%
Sodium 100mg	4%
Total Carbohydrate 5g	2%
Dietary Fiber 1g	4%
Sugars 2g	
Protein 21g	

SWORDFISH SHRIMP KABOBS

Number of Servings: 4

1 lb	Swordfish fillet	**2 Tbs**	Low sodium soy sauce
8	Large shrimp		
2 c	Tomatoes, wedged	**1/2 c**	White cooking wine
8	Medium mushrooms	**2 Tbs**	Lemon juice
1	Medium red onion, wedged	**1 Tbs**	Fresh lemon peel
		1 tsp	Garlic, minced
1/2	Yellow bell pepper, chunked	**1/4 c**	Extra virgin olive oil
1	Green bell pepper, chunked	**2 Tbs**	Dried dill weed

For the kabobs: on four metal or soaked wooden skewers, place the swordfish, tomato, shrimp, onion and peppers accordingly. Coat grill with nonstick cooking spray before starting grill. Grill kabobs, uncovered, over medium heat for 3 minutes, turning once. Baste with some of the reserved marinade. Grill 3-4 minutes or longer until fish flakes and shrimp turn pink, turning and basting frequently.

Marinade: Combine all other ingredients; blend well. Pour over fish kabobs and cover bowl. Let stand for at least 1 hour. Remove fish kabobs from marinade and cook according to recipe. Marinade may be used to baste fish while cooking.

Nutrition Facts

Serving Size 1 skewer (373g)
Servings Per Container 4

Amount Per Serving

Calories 370 Calories from Fat 170

	% Daily Value
Total Fat 19g	29%
Saturated Fat 3g	15%
Trans Fat 0g	
Cholesterol 65mg	22%
Sodium 345mg	14%
Total Carbohydrate 19g	6%
Dietary Fiber 3g	12%
Sugars 6g	
Protein 28g	

DAN'S SHRIMP AND SCALLOPS

Number of Servings: 8

16	Large shrimp	**1/2 c**	Green bell peppers, chopped
1 1/2 lbs	Scallops		
1/4 c	Light butter	**1**	Clove garlic
1 c	Fresh mushrooms, sliced	**1/4 c**	Lemon juice
		1/2 c	Capers, canned, drained
1/2 c	Green onions, tops and bulbs, chopped		

Preheat oven to 350°. Wash, clean and cut scallops into 1-inch pieces, if large and place in a roasting pan. Add shrimp and butter. Add mushrooms, onions, peppers, garlic and lemon juice. Top with capers. Bake for 20-30 minutes, turning once. Garnish with parsley, if desired. Serve over brown rice or whole wheat pasta.

 Submitted by Dr. Dan Wise

Nutrition Facts

Serving Size 3/4 cup (144g)
Servings Per Container 8

Amount Per Serving	
Calories 120	Calories from Fat 35

	% Daily Value
Total Fat 4g	6%
Saturated Fat 2g	10%
Trans Fat 0g	
Cholesterol 60mg	20%
Sodium 420mg	18%
Total Carbohydrate 4g	1%
Dietary Fiber 1g	4%
Sugars 1g	
Protein 18g	

When is it too hot to exercise outdoors? Use the 150 rule: If temperature plus humidity is greater than 150°, do not exercise or perform other vigorous activities outdoors. Exercise indoors where climate can be controlled.

SHRIMP CREOLE

Number of Servings: 8

2 Tbs	Whole wheat flour
2 Tbs	All purpose flour
1/2 c	Green onions, chopped
1 c	Celery, diced
4 Tbs	Extra virgin olive oil
1-1/2 c	Yellow onion, chopped
2/3 c	Green bell pepper, chopped
2	Garlic cloves
1	6 oz can no salt added tomato paste
16 oz	Tomatoes, chopped
8 oz	No salt added tomato sauce
1 c	Water
1 tsp	Ground black pepper
1/4 tsp	Cayenne pepper
2 tsp	Low sodium Worcestershire sauce
1 Tbs	Fresh lemon juice
1 tsp	Bay leaves
3 lbs	Medium shrimp
1/2 c	Parsley, chopped
3 c	Brown rice
1/4 tsp	Hot pepper sauce

Make a dark roux with the oil and flour by cooking the oil and flour over a low heat in a heavy pan. Stir constantly with a wooden spoon until the flour darkens, first to a golden brown and then, if you are patient, a dark coffee color. The aroma should be "nutty". This can take 30-40 minutes, don't be impatient and try to go fast as this will ruin the roux and the creole as well.

Add onions, green onions, celery, green pepper and garlic to the roux. Cook slowly until the vegetables are soft but not brown. Add the tomato sauce, tomatoes, tomato paste, water, pepper, hot sauce, cayenne, bay leaves, Worcestershire sauce and lemon juice.

Simmer very slowly for 1 hour or more covered. Add shrimp and cook until just done. This

SHRIMP CREOLE

continued

will only take a couple of minutes and should be done just before serving. Add parsley before serving. Serve over brown rice.

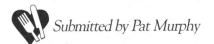

Submitted by Pat Murphy

Nutrition Facts

Serving Size 1/2 cup (465g)
Servings Per Container 8

Amount Per Serving	
Calories 400 Calories from Fat 100	
	% Daily Value
Total Fat 11g	17%
Saturated Fat 1.5g	8%
Trans Fat 0g	
Cholesterol 260mg	87%
Sodium 310mg	13%
Total Carbohydrate 36g	12%
Dietary Fiber 5g	20%
Sugars 8g	
Protein 39g	

To roast peppers, put whole peppers on the grill over medium heat for 15-20 minutes, turning occasionally until skin is charred on all sides. Put the peppers in a brown bag, fold over the top to seal, and cool for about 15 minutes. Then cut peppers lengthwise in half and discard stems and seeds; place cut-side down on work surface and scrape off skin with a small knife.

GRILLED SEA SCALLOPS

Number of Servings: 5

20 oz	Scallops, steamed (lightly poached)	**1/2 c**	Shallots, peeled and chopped
1 Tbs	Extra virgin olive oil	**1/2 c**	Water
1/8 c	Balsamic vinegar	**1 tsp**	Ground cumin
1 Tbs	Splenda® brown sugar blend	**1 tsp**	Ground chili pepper
1/2 tsp	White pepper	**1/2 tsp**	Minced garlic
1/2 tsp	Cayenne pepper	**1/4 c**	Water
4	Red bell peppers, diced	**1/2 tsp**	White pepper
		1 tsp	Apple cider vinegar
		3 tsp	Honey
		3 tsp	Fresh cilantro, diced

Place olive oil, balsamic vinegar, Splenda® brown sugar blend, 1/2 teaspoon white pepper and cayenne pepper in a medium bowl. Mix well using a whisk. Add steamed scallops to marinade and let sit for a minimum of half an hour.

Sauté peppers and shallots together in a nonstick sauté pan coated with cooking spray. Add 1/2 cup water and simmer 20 minutes or until peppers are soft; drain any water left in pan.

Nutrition Facts

Serving Size 1 cup (195g)
Servings Per Container 5

Amount Per Serving

Calories 150   Calories from Fat 35

	% Daily Value
Total Fat 3.5g	5%
Saturated Fat 0.5g	3%
Trans Fat 0g	
Cholesterol 20mg	7%
Sodium 100mg	4%
Total Carbohydrate 17g	6%
Dietary Fiber 2g	8%
Sugars 10g	
Protein 10g	

To prepare the sweet pepper and cilantro coulis: place peppers, shallots, cumin, chili pepper, garlic, 1/4 cup water, white pepper, apple cider vinegar and honey in a food processor. Blend until smooth. Add cilantro and set aside.

Grill scallops on hot gas or charcoal grill, only 1 minute per side. Ladle coulis onto serving plates. Arrange grilled scallops over coulis and garnish with steamed shoestring vegetables, if desired.

CLAM FRITTERS

Number of Servings: 6

6-1/2 oz	Minced clams		**1/2 c**	Whole wheat flour
3 Tbs	White onion, chopped		**1**	Fresh eggplant
1/2 tsp	Salt substitute		**1**	Omega-3 egg, beaten
1 tsp	Canola oil		**1**	Jalapeno pepper
2 Tbs	Skim milk		**1/8 tsp**	Ground black pepper
1 tsp	Baking powder			

Peel and cube the eggplant. Place in a saucepan with 1/3 cup water, cover and cook until tender. Drain and mash. Drain the clams and blend with the eggplant. Reserve clam juice. Stir in the egg, onion, peppers, salt and pepper. Mix the flour and baking powder and slowly blend with the eggplant mixture adding enough milk to make a drop batter. You may use the reserved clam juice if you prefer. Fry in a nonstick fry pan until well browned using about 1/3 cup of batter for each fritter. Drain on paper towels and serve hot. The peppers can be added to each individual fritter or to just part of the mix.

Nutrition Facts

Serving Size 1 fritter (155g)
Servings Per Container 6

Amount Per Serving

Calories 90   Calories from Fat 15

	% Daily Value
Total Fat 2g	3%
Saturated Fat 0g	0%
Trans Fat 0g	
Cholesterol 35mg	12%
Sodium 270mg	11%
Total Carbohydrate 14g	5%
Dietary Fiber 4g	16%
Sugars 3g	
Protein 6g	

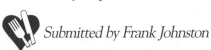

Submitted by Frank Johnston

KATHY'S CHICKEN SQUASH PASTA MEDLEY

Number of Servings: 5

5	Boneless skinless chicken breasts, cut into strips
1 tsp	Salt substitute
2 tsp	Minced garlic
2 Tbs	Extra virgin olive oil
2 c	Zucchini, sliced
2 c	Yellow squash, sliced
1 c	White onion, chopped
1/2 tsp	Garlic powder
1/2 tsp	Ground black pepper
16 oz	Whole wheat penne pasta

Season the chicken with salt substitute and 1 teaspoon garlic. Heat the oil in a sauté pan over medium-high heat. Add the chicken strips. In a separate sauté pan, combine zucchini, yellow squash, onion, garlic powder, pepper and remaining garlic; cook until semi soft. Mushrooms or your favorite veggies can be added. Combine all the above and serve over whole wheat penne pasta.

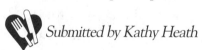 *Submitted by Kathy Heath*

Nutrition Facts

Serving Size 1-1/2 cups (340g)
Servings Per Container 5

Amount Per Serving	
Calories 560	Calories from Fat 90

	% Daily Value
Total Fat 10g	15%
Saturated Fat 1g	5%
Trans Fat 0g	
Cholesterol 70mg	23%
Sodium 100mg	4%
Total Carbohydrate 75g	25%
Dietary Fiber 10g	40%
Sugars 6g	
Protein 40g	

Summer squash, including zucchini, yellow squash and pattypan, can be cut into chunks and used for kabobs. You can also slice them lengthwise.

CITRUS CRUNCH CHICKEN

Number of Servings: 4

1	Lemon	**1 lb**	Boneless skinless chicken breasts
1	Lime	**3/4 c**	Seasoned bread crumbs
1	Orange		

Preheat oven to 400°. Grate peel from half of each of the fruits; combine with the bread crumbs. Coat chicken evenly with the bread crumb mixture. Cut fruit into thin slices; arrange, with slices slightly overlapping, on bottom of foil-lined or parchment-lined 13x9-inch baking pan. Top with chicken. Bake 30 minutes or until chicken is cooked through. Serve with the fruit slices.

Nutrition Facts

Serving Size 3 oz breast (200g)
Servings Per Container 4

Amount Per Serving

Calories 240   Calories from Fat 25

	% Daily Value
Total Fat 2.5g	4%
Saturated Fat 0.5g	3%
Trans Fat 0g	
Cholesterol 65mg	22%
Sodium 470mg	20%
Total Carbohydrate 22g	7%
Dietary Fiber 3g	12%
Sugars 5g	
Protein 30g	

SPICY CHICKEN BARBEQUE

Number of Servings: 6

1/4 c	White onion, chopped	**3 tsp**	Splenda®
2 tsp	Minced garlic	**2 tsp**	Dry mustard
2 Tbs	Canola oil	**1/2 tsp**	Ground black pepper
1/2 c	Low sodium ketchup	**1 tsp**	Hot pepper sauce
2/3 c	White vinegar	**3 lbs**	Skinless bone-in
2 Tbs	Fresh lemon juice		chicken breasts
2 Tbs	Worcestershire sauce		

In a medium saucepan, cook onion and garlic in oil until tender. Stir in all other ingredients. Cover and simmer for 30 minutes stirring occasionally. Place chicken in large dish. Pour onion mixture over chicken. Marinate chicken breasts for at least 3 hours. Preheat grill. Grill, bake or broil chicken for 20 minutes; flip chicken breast and continue to cook 20 minutes longer. Brush chicken with sauce often.

Nutrition Facts

Serving Size 3 oz breast (297g)
Servings Per Container 6

Amount Per Serving	
Calories 340 Calories from Fat 70	
	% Daily Value
Total Fat 8g	12%
Saturated Fat 1g	5%
Trans Fat 0g	
Cholesterol 130mg	43%
Sodium 230mg	10%
Total Carbohydrate 9g	3%
Dietary Fiber 1g	4%
Sugars 6g	
Protein 53g	

To save money, combine a bit of nonfat dry milk with low fat liquid milk. Keep in the refrigerator and shake just before using.

TURKEY CACCIATORE BURGERS ON PORTABELLA "BUNS"

Number of Servings: 4

1/3 c	Yellow onion, chopped	**6**	Crimini mushrooms, chopped
1 tsp	Extra virgin olive oil	**1/2**	Red bell pepper, chopped
1 tsp	Crushed chili pepper flakes	**2 tsp**	Garlic, minced
3 Tbs	No salt added tomato paste	**1 Tbs**	Low sodium Worcestershire sauce
2 c	Arugula, chopped	**4**	Portabella mushrooms
1/2 c	Light parmesan cheese, grated	**1/3 c**	White onion, chopped
1-1/3 lb	99% fat free ground turkey	**1/2 c**	Fresh parsley, chopped

Preheat oven to 450°. Combine meat with a dash of salt and pepper, crimini mushrooms, pepper, onion, garlic, tomato paste, Worcestershire, red pepper flakes, cheese and parsley. Score and form meat into 4 large patties, 1-inch thick. Drizzle extra virgin olive oil on top of the patties. Heat a large nonstick skillet over medium heat. Fry patties for 5-6 minutes on each side.

Nutrition Facts

Serving Size 1 burger (361g)
Servings Per Container 4

Amount Per Serving	
Calories 310	Calories from Fat 60

	% Daily Value
Total Fat 7g	11%
Saturated Fat 0g	0%
Trans Fat 0g	
Cholesterol 75mg	25%
Sodium 340mg	14%
Total Carbohydrate 20g	7%
Dietary Fiber 3g	12%
Sugars 6g	
Protein 44g	

Place portabella caps on a small baking sheet grill side up and drizzle extra virgin olive oil on them. Roast caps 12 minutes. Remove from oven and season with salt and pepper. Top each cap with about 1/2 cup arugula and a burger. Top with onions and tomatoes and serve.

ANGELA'S BBQ

Number of Servings: 10

4 lb	Lean pork tenderloin	**2 Tbs**	Low sodium barbecue sauce
3/4 c	Low sodium barbecue sauce	**1 Tbs**	Mustard
4 c	Cabbage, chopped	**10**	Whole wheat hamburger buns
3/4 c	Light mayonnaise		
1/4 c	Low sodium ketchup	**1/2 tsp**	Ground black pepper

Pork: Place 4 lbs of pork tenderloin in a crock pot with enough water to cover meat. Add 3/4 cup barbeque sauce and pepper. Cook for 6-8 hours on low in crock pot. Remove tenderloin and grind in a food processor.

Slaw: Combine mayonnaise, ketchup, 2 tablespoons barbeque sauce and mustard; mix well. If desired, add additional amounts of ketchup, barbeque sauce and mustard to taste. Add mixture to chopped cabbage and toss to blend.

Add slaw to both sides of whole wheat buns. Add 3 ounces cooked pork barbeque to hamburger bun. Toast sandwich in a nonstick skillet.

Nutrition Facts

Serving Size 1 sandwich (307g)
Servings Per Container 10

Amount Per Serving

Calories 410 Calories from Fat 130

	% Daily Value
Total Fat 14g	22%
Saturated Fat 2.5g	13%
Trans Fat 0g	
Cholesterol 125mg	42%
Sodium 490mg	20%
Total Carbohydrate 29g	10%
Dietary Fiber 4g	16%
Sugars 7g	
Protein 42g	

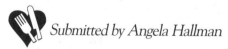

Submitted by Angela Hallman

SWEET SMOKEY BARBEQUE SAUCE

Number of Servings: 12

2 tsp	Canola oil	**3 Tbs**	Worcestershire sauce
1 tsp	Garlic, minced	**1/3 c**	Splenda
1 c	White onion, minced	**2 tsp**	Molasses
6 oz	No salt added tomato paste	**1 tsp**	Ground chili pepper
		1 tsp	Dry mustard
1 c	Water	**1/4 tsp**	Hot pepper sauce
2 Tbs	Apple cider vinegar		

In a medium saucepan, heat oil and garlic over medium heat for 1 minute. Add onion and cook for 10 minutes, until onion is soft and translucent. You can put onion mixture into food processor and puree if you don't want small onion chunks in the sauce.

Add the remaining ingredients, stir well and simmer for 20 minutes over low heat.
Remove from heat and place in blender; grind to smooth and blend flavors. Cool, cover and refrigerate. Keeps for 2 weeks.

Nutrition Facts

Serving Size 2 tablespoons (57g)
Servings Per Container 12

Amount Per Serving	
Calories 35	Calories from Fat 10

	% Daily Value
Total Fat 1g	2%
Saturated Fat 0g	0%
Trans Fat 0g	
Cholesterol 0mg	0%
Sodium 60mg	3%
Total Carbohydrate 7g	2%
Dietary Fiber 1g	4%
Sugars 3g	
Protein 1g	

ASPARAGUS WITH SESAME SEEDS

Number of Servings: 2

1/2 lb Asparagus
2 Tbs Water
1 tsp Low sodium soy sauce
1 tsp Extra virgin olive oil

1/8 tsp Salt
1/8 tsp Ground black pepper
1 tsp Sesame seeds, toasted

Place asparagus in a steamer basket; place in a saucepan of 1-inch of water. Bring to a boil; cover and steam for 4-5 minutes or until crisp-tender. Transfer to a serving dish. In a small bowl, combine water, soy sauce, oil, salt and pepper; drizzle over asparagus. Sprinkle with toasted sesame seeds.

Nutrition Facts

Serving Size 1 cup (135g)
Servings Per Container 2

Amount Per Serving	
Calories 60	Calories from Fat 30

	% Daily Value
Total Fat 3.5g	5%
Saturated Fat 0g	0%
Trans Fat 0g	
Cholesterol 0mg	0%
Sodium 240mg	10%
Total Carbohydrate 5g	2%
Dietary Fiber 3g	12%
Sugars 2g	
Protein 3g	

VINAIGRETTE COLESLAW

Number of Servings: 4

3 c	Cabbage, shredded	**3 tsp**	Splenda®
2 Tbs	Red bell peppers, chopped	**2 tsp**	Dijon mustard
		2 tsp	Extra virgin olive oil
2 Tbs	Parsley, chopped	**1/4 tsp**	Fresh basil, minced
2 Tbs	Green onion, chopped	**1/2 tsp**	Ground black pepper
6 Tbs	Cider vinegar	**1/4 tsp**	Garlic herb Mrs. Dash®
2 Tbs	Water		

In a small bowl, combine the cabbage, red pepper, parsley and onion. In another bowl, combine the remaining ingredients; pour over cabbage mixture and toss to coat. Cover and refrigerate until chilled. Toss before serving.

Nutrition Facts

Serving Size 3/4 cup (102g)
Servings Per Container 4

Amount Per Serving	
Calories 45	Calories from Fat 20

	% Daily Value
Total Fat 2.5g	4%
Saturated Fat 0g	0%
Trans Fat 0g	
Cholesterol 0mg	0%
Sodium 45mg	2%
Total Carbohydrate 6g	2%
Dietary Fiber 2g	8%
Sugars 4g	
Protein 1g	

WHOLE WHEAT CARROT MUFFINS

Number of Servings: 6

1/2 c	Whole wheat flour	**1/4 c**	Trans fat free margarine
2 Tbs	Whole wheat flour	**2 Tbs**	Orange juice
1/4 c	Brown sugar, packed	**1**	Omega-3 egg, beaten
1/2 tsp	Cinnamon	**3/4 c**	Carrots, grated
1/2 tsp	Baking powder	**1/4 c**	Raisins
1/4 tsp	Baking soda		
1/4 tsp	Salt substitute		

Preheat oven to 350°. In a bowl, combine the flour, brown sugar, cinnamon, baking powder, baking soda and salt substitute. In a small mixing bowl, beat the margarine, orange juice and only 2 tablespoons of the egg on medium speed for 1 minute (mixture will not be smooth). Pour into dry ingredients; stir just until blended. Fold in carrots and raisins.

Nutrition Facts

Serving Size 1 muffin (66g)
Servings Per Container 6

Amount Per Serving

Calories 190   Calories from Fat 80

	% Daily Value
Total Fat 9g	14%
Saturated Fat 1.5g	8%
Trans Fat 0g	
Cholesterol 30mg	10%
Sodium 300mg	13%
Total Carbohydrate 25g	8%
Dietary Fiber 2g	8%
Sugars 15g	
Protein 3g	

Coat muffin cups with nonstick cooking spray or use paper liners; fill half full with batter. Bake for 20-25 minutes or until a toothpick comes out clean. Cool for 5 minutes before removing from pan to a wire rack.

BLUEBERRY GELATIN SALAD

Number of Servings: 9

1-1/2 c Fresh blueberries
16 oz Canned crushed pineapple, light syrup, with juice
2 Small boxes sugar free wild berry gelatin
2 c Water

8 oz Fat free cream cheese, room temperature
1/2 c Splenda®
1 tsp Vanilla extract
1/2 c Pecans, chopped

Dissolve gelatin with 2 cups boiling water in a 9x11-inch pan. Add pineapple with juice and blueberries to gelatin mixture. Refrigerate for approximately 2 hours. In a separate bowl combine cream cheese, Splenda®, vanilla and pecans; spread evenly over gelatin mixture. Refrigerate.

 Submitted by Kathy Jones

Nutrition Facts	
Serving Size 1/2 cup (161g)	
Servings Per Container 9	
Amount Per Serving	
Calories 120 Calories from Fat 45	
	% Daily Value
Total Fat 5g	8%
Saturated Fat 0.5g	3%
Trans Fat 0g	
Cholesterol 0mg	0%
Sodium 150mg	6%
Total Carbohydrate 14g	5%
Dietary Fiber 2g	8%
Sugars 9g	
Protein 5g	

PEACH CRISP

Number of Servings: 4

2 c	Fresh peeled peaches, sliced	**1 Tbs**	Brown sugar
1/2 tsp	Ground cinnamon	**1 Tbs**	Trans fat free margarine
1/2 tsp	Ground nutmeg	**2 c**	Low fat no sugar
1/2 c	Old fashioned oats		added vanilla ice cream
1 Tbs	All purpose flour		

Preheat oven to 350°. Combine peaches, 1/4 teaspoon cinnamon and nutmeg in a large bowl; stir well. Spoon into 8x8-inch dish sprayed with cooking spray; set aside. In another bowl, combine oats, remaining 1/4 teaspoon cinnamon, flour and sugar; stir well. Cut in margarine with a pastry blender or fork until mixture resembles coarse meal; sprinkle evenly over the peach mixture.
Bake for 40 minutes or until lightly browned. Serve warm over low fat no sugar added ice cream.

Nutrition Facts

Serving Size 1/2 cup (174g)
Servings Per Container 4

Amount Per Serving

Calories 220   Calories from Fat 70

	% Daily Value
Total Fat 8g	12%
Saturated Fat 3.5g	18%
Trans Fat 0g	
Cholesterol 10mg	3%
Sodium 70mg	3%
Total Carbohydrate 36g	13%
Dietary Fiber 3g	12%
Sugars 14g	
Protein 5g	

BLACKBERRY PEACH CRISP

Number of Servings: 4

1 c	Blackberries		**2 Tbs**	Brown sugar
1 c	Peaches, sliced		**4 tsp**	Canola oil
4 tsp	Orange juice		**1 tsp**	Honey
1/2 tsp	Vanilla extract		**1 tsp**	Ground cinnamon
3 Tbs	Whole wheat flour		**1/8 tsp**	Ground nutmeg
3 Tbs	Old fashioned oats			

Heat oven to 375°. Coat four 4-oz ramekins with nonstick cooking spray. Combine berries, peaches, juice and vanilla in a bowl and mix well. Spoon 1/4 portion of fruit into each ramekin. In a separate bowl, combine remaining ingredients with hands until moist and crumbly. Then spoon crumble mixture evenly over the top of fruit. Bake 15-20 minutes or until fruit bubbles and top is golden brown.

Nutrition Facts

Serving Size 1/2 cup (89g)
Servings Per Container 4

Amount Per Serving	
Calories 140	Calories from Fat 45

	% Daily Value
Total Fat 5g	8%
Saturated Fat 0g	0%
Trans Fat 0g	
Cholesterol 0mg	0%
Sodium 0mg	0%
Total Carbohydrate 22g	7%
Dietary Fiber 4g	16%
Sugars 10g	
Protein 2g	

Many vegetables and fruits, including potatoes and apples, retain many of their nutrients in their skin. So when possible, leave the skin on your fruits and vegetables and cook them whole.

JORDAN'S BERRY BANANA SMOOTHIE

Number of Servings: 2

6	Fresh strawberries		**1 c**	Soy milk
1	Small banana		**6-10**	Ice cubes
6 oz	Nonfat vanilla yogurt, sweetened with Splenda®			

In an electric blender, blend ingredients with ice and serve. Optional: 1/2 cup cooked oatmeal for fiber. Skim milk can be substituted for soy milk. Be creative and try different types of fruit.

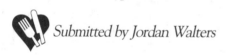 *Submitted by Jordan Walters*

Nutrition Facts

Serving Size 12 ounces (303g)
Servings Per Container 2

Amount Per Serving	
Calories 150 Calories from Fat 25	
	% Daily Value
Total Fat 2.5g	4%
Saturated Fat 0g	0%
Trans Fat 0g	
Cholesterol 0mg	0%
Sodium 120mg	5%
Total Carbohydrate 26g	9%
Dietary Fiber 4g	16%
Sugars 15g	
Protein 10g	

STRAWBERRY PIE

Number of Servings: 8

1	Small box sugar free strawberry gelatin	**8 oz**	Fat free whipped topping
1/4 c	Hot water	**1**	9" reduced fat graham cracker pie crust
16 oz	Low fat strawberry yogurt		

In a bowl, combine hot water and gelatin to dissolve. Let cool and add yogurt. Add cool whip to gelatin/yogurt mixture and mix. Pour into graham cracker crust. Garnish with strawberries. Refrigerate.

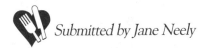 *Submitted by Jane Neely*

Nutrition Facts

Serving Size 1/8 slice (83g)
Servings Per Container 8

Amount Per Serving

Calories 110   Calories from Fat 5

% Daily Value

Total Fat 1g	2%
Saturated Fat 0g	0%
Trans Fat 0g	
Cholesterol 0mg	0%
Sodium 200mg	8%
Total Carbohydrate 16g	5%
Dietary Fiber 0g	0%
Sugars 9g	
Protein 5g	

Almonds:
- *After opening, almonds will keep 4 to 6 months under refrigeration.*
- *Opened nuts, if frozen, will keep for 9 to 12 months.*
- *To toast almonds, spread in a single layer on a baking pan and bake at 300-350°F for 8-10 minutes, stirring occasionally until almonds darken slightly (they will continue to brown slightly when removed from the oven).*

STRAWBERRY ANGEL FOOD DELIGHT

Number of Servings: 8

1 Sugar free angel food cake

4 c Whole strawberries

1 Box sugar free instant vanilla pudding

2 c Fat free whipped topping

Cut cake in half horizontally. In a food processor or blender, process strawberries until almost pureed (puree has bits of strawberries).

Place pureed strawberries in a medium mixing bowl and stir in pudding mix. Place bottom half of cake on plate and spread a layer of strawberry mixture over it. Place upper portion of cake on the bottom half. Fold in 2 cups of fat free whipped topping with remaining strawberry mixture and spread over the entire cake. Add sliced strawberries and blueberries, as a garnish on top of cake.

Nutrition Facts	
Serving Size 2-inch slice (121g)	
Servings Per Container 8	
Amount Per Serving	
Calories 110	Calories from Fat 0
	% Daily Value
Total Fat 0g	0%
Saturated Fat 0g	0%
Trans Fat 0g	
Cholesterol 0mg	0%
Sodium 170mg	7%
Total Carbohydrate 23g	8%
Dietary Fiber 1g	4%
Sugars 0g	
Protein 2g	

CHERRY CHOCOLATE CAKE

Number of Servings: 12

1/3 c	Sugar	**1/2 c**	Splenda®
1/2 c	Unsweetened cocoa powder	**1/2 tsp**	Cream of tartar
2-1/2 c	Cake flour	**1 tsp**	Almond extract
1 tsp	Baking soda	**3**	Egg whites
2 tsp	Baking powder	**2**	20 oz cans no sugar added cherry pie filling
1/2 tsp	Ground cinnamon	**3/4 tsp**	Powdered sugar
1/4 tsp	Salt substitute		

Preheat oven to 350°. In a mixing bowl, combine the dry ingredients except powdered sugar. Stir in eggs and almond extract. Add one can of pie filling and stir until blended. Transfer to a 13x9-inch baking pan coated with nonstick cooking spray. Bake for 30-35 minutes or until toothpick comes out clean. Cool completely. Dust with powdered sugar. Top individual servings with remaining pie filling.

Nutrition Facts

Serving Size 2-inch square (143g)
Servings Per Container 12

Amount Per Serving	
Calories 160	Calories from Fat 5

	% Daily Value
Total Fat 0.5g	1%
Saturated Fat 0g	0%
Trans Fat 0g	
Cholesterol 0mg	0%
Sodium 300mg	13%
Total Carbohydrate 28g	9%
Dietary Fiber 1g	4%
Sugars 7g	
Protein 9g	

KEY LIME PIE

Number of Servings: 8

2	Low fat key lime pie yogurt	**1 c**	Water
1	Graham cracker pie crust	**1**	Large box sugar free lime gelatin
8 oz	Fat free whipped topping		

Boil one cup water and add it to gelatin mix. Combine remainder of ingredients and pour into graham cracker crust. Refrigerate until firm.

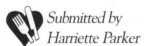 *Submitted by Harriette Parker*

Nutrition Facts

Serving Size 1/8 slice (143g)
Servings Per Container 8

Amount Per Serving

Calories 210   Calories from Fat 10

	% Daily Value
Total Fat 1g	2%
Saturated Fat 0g	0%
Trans Fat 0g	
Cholesterol 5mg	2%
Sodium 100mg	29%
Total Carbohydrate 21g	7%
Dietary Fiber 0g	0%
Sugars 11g	
Protein 12g	

To make fat free broth, chill your meat or chicken broth. The fat will rise to the top and you can remove it before using the broth.

KEY LIME-COCONUT MINI CHEESECAKES

Number of Servings: 14

14	Reduced fat vanilla wafers	**1/2 tsp**	Vanilla extract
8 oz	Fat free cream cheese	**1/4 tsp**	Coconut extract
8 oz	Low fat cream cheese	**1/2 c**	Fat free sour cream
1/2 c	Splenda®	**1 Tbs**	Sugar
1/4 c	Sugar	**2-1/3 Tbs**	Dried coconut, toasted
1/2 c	Egg substitute	**1**	Lime zest
1 tsp	Key lime juice		

Preheat oven to 350°. Place 14 paper baking cups in muffin pans and coat lightly with cooking spray. Place 1 vanilla wafer in each baking cup.

Beat together cream cheeses, Splenda® and sugar at medium speed with a mixer until smooth. Add egg substitute and next 3 ingredients, beating until smooth. Spoon mixture evenly into baking cups.

Bake 10-12 minutes or until set. Remove pans from oven. Stir together sour cream and 1 tablespoon sugar. Spread 1 teaspoon sour cream mixture over top of each cheesecake (sour cream mixture will not completely cover each top). Cool on a wire rack for 15 minutes. Cover and chill for at least 2 hours. Before serving, sprinkle tops evenly with coconut and lime zest.

Nutrition Facts

Serving Size 1 mini cheesecake (67g)
Servings Per Container 14

Amount Per Serving

Calories 110   Calories from Fat 35

	% Daily Value
Total Fat 3.5g	5%
Saturated Fat 2g	10%
Trans Fat 0g	
Cholesterol 10mg	3%
Sodium 180mg	8%
Total Carbohydrate 13g	4%
Dietary Fiber 0g	0%
Sugars 7g	
Protein 6g	

MEME'S SQUASH PIE

Number of Servings: 8

3 c	Yellow squash, sliced	**1 tsp**	Vanilla extract
1 c	Evaporated skim milk	**1/2 tsp**	Salt substitute
4	Omega-3 eggs	**1 Tbs**	All purpose flour
3/4 c	Splenda®		

Preheat oven to 350°. In a microwave safe bowl, cook yellow squash pieces until very tender. Drain. Stir cooked squash until pieces are broken up. Add all remaining ingredients. Stir until mixed well. Pour into two greased 9-inch pie plates. Bake for 30 minutes.

 Submitted by Ruth Wagoner

Nutrition Facts

Serving Size 2-inch wedge (103g)
Servings Per Container 8

Amount Per Serving

Calories 80   Calories from Fat 20

% Daily Value

Total Fat 2g	3%
Saturated Fat 0.5g	3%
Trans Fat 0g	
Cholesterol 90mg	30%
Sodium 40mg	2%
Total Carbohydrate 8g	3%
Dietary Fiber 0g	0%
Sugars 5g	
Protein 6g	

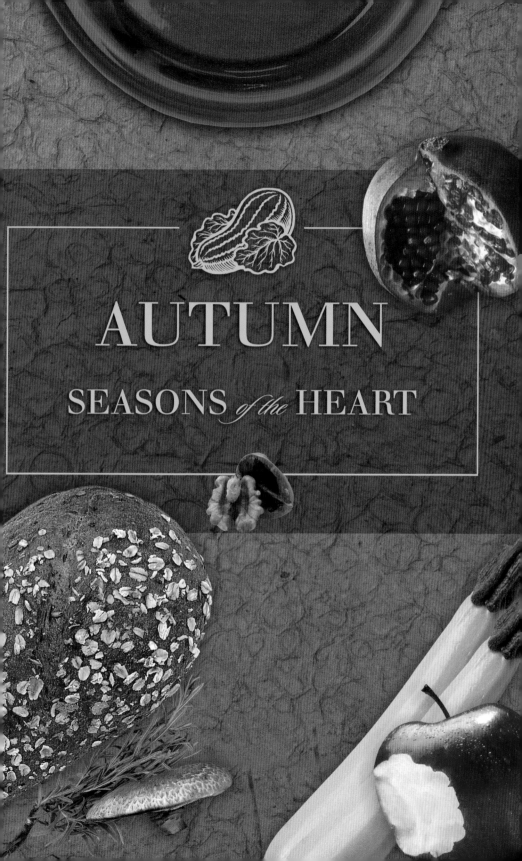

AUTUMN

SEASONS *of the* HEART

7 LAYER DIP

Number of Servings: 48

1	15 oz can fat free refried beans	**1 c**	Low fat four cheese Mexican blend, finely shredded
1 Tbs	Taco seasoning	**1/2 c**	Green onions, tops and bulbs, chopped
1 c	Fat free sour cream	**2 Tbs**	Black olives without pits, sliced
1 c	Chunky salsa		
1 c	Green leaf lettuce, shredded		

Mix beans and taco seasoning mix. Spread onto bottom of 9-inch pie plate. Layer all remaining ingredients over bean mixture; cover. Refrigerate several hours or until chilled. Serve with natural tortilla chips.

Nutrition Facts

Serving Size 2 tablespoons (25g)
Servings Per Container 48

Amount Per Serving

Calories 20   Calories from Fat 5

% Daily Value

Total Fat 0.5g	1%
Saturated Fat 0g	0%
Trans Fat 0g	
Cholesterol 0mg	0%
Sodium 115mg	5%
Total Carbohydrate 3g	1%
Dietary Fiber 1g	4%
Sugars 1g	
Protein 1g	

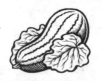

ELAINE'S HOM-MOS BI-TAHINI

Number of Servings: 32

1	15 oz can garbanzo beans	**1 tsp**	Salt substitute
2	Fresh garlic cloves	**1/2 c**	Extra virgin olive oil
2 Tbs	Tahini sesame seed paste	**1/2 c**	Fresh lemon juice
		1/2 tsp	Ground cumin

Combine above ingredients in blender and process at high speed for 2-3 minutes until smooth. Add extra lemon juice and salt substitute, if desired. Pour into small bowl and garnish lightly with parsley, paprika or cumin and serve. Serve with whole wheat pita chips or crackers, if desired.

Submitted by Elaine Barnes

Nutrition Facts

Serving Size 1 tablespoon (22g)
Servings Per Container 32

Amount Per Serving

Calories 50 Calories from Fat 35

	% Daily Value
Total Fat 4g	6%
Saturated Fat 0.5g	3%
Trans Fat 0g	
Cholesterol 0mg	0%
Sodium 40mg	2%
Total Carbohydrate 3g	1%
Dietary Fiber 1g	4%
Sugars 0g	
Protein 1g	

Hummus is popular in various local forms throughout the Arab world. In the Middle East, the age and quality of a family's hummus recipe is a sign of social status. Connoisseurs can easily and accurately identify a family's lineage simply based on the household's daily hummus.

CHICKEN BROCCOLI CHOWDER

Number of Servings: 6

1/2 c	Onion, chopped	**1**	10 3/4 oz can 98% fat free 30% reduced sodium cream of chicken soup
10 oz	Frozen chopped broccoli, cooked, drained		
2 c	Carrots, sliced	**1/2 c**	Whole grain oat flour
2 c	Water	**2 c**	Skim milk
9 oz	Boneless skinless chicken breasts, diced	**3 oz**	Low fat Swiss cheese, shredded

Combine onion, broccoli, carrots, water, chicken and chicken soup in a 4-qt saucepan or Dutch oven. Bring to a boil over medium-high heat; reduce heat. Cover; simmer about 10 minutes. Bring to a full rolling boil; gradually add oat flour, stirring constantly. Stir in milk. Simmer, stirring occasionally, about 10 minutes. Remove from heat; stir in cheese. Cover; let stand 3-5 minutes before serving. Sprinkle with Savory Add-A-Crunch to serve (Autumn pg. 176).

Note: Additional milk may be added if soup becomes too thick upon standing.

Nutrition Facts

Serving Size 1 cup (378g)
Servings Per Container 6

Amount Per Serving	
Calories 180	Calories from Fat 30

	% Daily Value
Total Fat 3g	5%
Saturated Fat 1g	5%
Trans Fat 0g	
Cholesterol 30mg	10%
Sodium 390mg	16%
Total Carbohydrate 20g	7%
Dietary Fiber 4g	16%
Sugars 8g	
Protein 20g	

SANTA FE SOUP

Number of Servings: 16

1	Yellow onion, chopped	**16 oz**	No salt added pinto beans
2 lbs	99% fat free ground turkey	**2 c**	Tomatoes, wedged
1 oz	Dry ranch salad dressing mix	**2 c**	Water
		16 oz	Frozen corn
1 oz	30% less sodium taco seasoning mix	**16 oz**	No salt added diced tomatoes
2 c	Dry black beans	**3 oz**	Green chili peppers
16 oz	No salt added kidney beans		

Prepare dried black beans as directed on package to hydrate. Cook meat and onion together until meat is browned. Stir ranch style dressing mix and taco seasoning mix into meat. Add remaining ingredients with juices from all except black beans. Add water. Simmer for two hours. If mixture is too thick, add additional water. Garnish each serving with fat free sour cream, 2% shredded cheddar cheese and sliced green onions, if desired. Serve with natural tortilla chips.

Nutrition Facts

Serving Size 1 cup (265g)
Servings Per Container 16

Amount Per Serving

Calories 270   Calories from Fat 10

	% Daily Value
Total Fat 1g	2%
Saturated Fat 0g	0%
Trans Fat 0g	
Cholesterol 20mg	7%
Sodium 360mg	15%
Total Carbohydrate 33g	11%
Dietary Fiber 7g	28%
Sugars 5g	
Protein 23g	

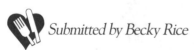 *Submitted by Becky Rice*

JAN'S TOMATO BASIL SOUP

Number of Servings: 10

1	46 oz can no salt added tomato juice
1/8 tsp	Baking soda
1 c	Fat free half and half
1	6 oz can no salt added tomato paste

1/2 tsp	Ground basil
1/2 tsp	Ground black pepper
1/2 tsp	Ground sage
1 Tbs	Cornstarch

Combine first seven ingredients in a large pot and stir to mix thoroughly. Heat to a boil; then simmer for 15 minutes. Then remove 1/2 cup of soup; place in a small bowl. Add 1 tablespoon cornstarch. With a fork whisk mixture until smooth. Add to pot; simmer for 15-20 minutes.

Submitted by Jan Wagoner

Nutrition Facts

Serving Size 1 cup (224g)
Servings Per Container 10

Amount Per Serving	
Calories 70	Calories from Fat 5

	% Daily Value
Total Fat 0.5g	1%
Saturated Fat 0g	0%
Trans Fat 0g	
Cholesterol 0mg	0%
Sodium 95mg	4%
Total Carbohydrate 14g	5%
Dietary Fiber 2g	8%
Sugars 9g	
Protein 3g	

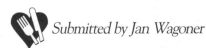

Tomatoes get their vivid red color from a powerful antioxidant called lycopene.

SPINACH SALAD

Number of Servings: 6

3/4 lb Fresh baby spinach
6 White mushrooms, trimmed and sliced
1/3 c Turkey bacon, cooked and crumbled

1 tsp Ground black pepper
3 Tbs Red wine vinegar
2 Tbs Extra virgin olive oil

Wash and dry the spinach. Combine spinach and mushrooms in a large serving bowl and set them aside (or refrigerate up to 6 hours).

In a skillet, over medium heat, add bacon and cook for approximately 5 minutes or until bacon just starts to get crisp. Don't let the bacon get too crisp or brown. While the bacon is cooking, season the salad with pepper. Remove cooked bacon from skillet and set on paper towels to soak up fat. Pour the vinegar into the skillet and bring the liquid in the skillet to a quick boil. Immediately pour the hot dressing over the spinach and toss well. Drizzle the olive oil over the salad and toss to mix. Add bacon pieces. Taste and add pepper, vinegar or oil if you like. Serve immediately.

Nutrition Facts	
Serving Size 1 cup (88g)	
Servings Per Container 6	
Amount Per Serving	
Calories 90	Calories from Fat 50
	% Daily Value
Total Fat 6g	9%
Saturated Fat 1g	5%
Trans Fat 0g	
Cholesterol 5mg	2%
Sodium 200mg	8%
Total Carbohydrate 7g	2%
Dietary Fiber 3g	12%
Sugars 0g	
Protein 3g	

HEARTY OATMEAL PANCAKES

Number of Servings: 4

1 c	Old fashioned oats	**1/4 tsp**	Salt substitute
1/4 c	All purpose flour	**1**	Omega-3 egg
3/4 c	Whole wheat flour	**2 c**	Low fat buttermilk
1 Tbs	Splenda®	**1 Tbs**	Canola oil
1 tsp	Baking powder	**1/2 Tbs**	Vanilla extract
1/2 tsp	Baking soda		

In a bowl, combine the first seven ingredients. In another bowl, combine the egg, buttermilk, oil and vanilla; mix well. Stir into the dry ingredients just until moistened. Pour batter by 1/4 cupful onto a hot griddle that has been coated with nonstick cooking spray. Turn when bubbles form on top; cook until the second side is golden brown. Serve with berries if desired.

Nutrition Facts

Serving Size 3 – 4-inch pancakes (196g)
Servings Per Container 4

Amount Per Serving	
Calories 310 Calories from Fat 70	
	% Daily Value
Total Fat 8g	12%
Saturated Fat 1.5g	8%
Trans Fat 0g	
Cholesterol 55mg	18%
Sodium 430mg	18%
Total Carbohydrate 46g	15%
Dietary Fiber 5g	20%
Sugars 7g	
Protein 13g	

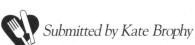 *Submitted by Kate Brophy*

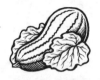

BALSAMIC GLAZED GRILLED SALMON

Number of Servings: 4

1/4 c	Balsamic vinegar
2 Tbs	Fresh lemon juice
2 Tbs	Brown sugar, packed

1 1/4 lbs Wild Alaskan salmon fillets

Preheat grill to medium heat. Whisk together vinegar, lemon juice and brown sugar in a small bowl; pour most of mixture over salmon. Place salmon fillets on a grill rack coated with nonstick cooking spray. Grill, covered with grill lid, over medium heat for 4-6 minutes (longer for salmon steaks) on each side or until fish flakes with a fork, basting occasionally with remaining mixture.

Nutrition Facts

Serving Size 5 ounce fillet (171g)
Servings Per Container 4

Amount Per Serving	
Calories 290 Calories from Fat 130	
	% Daily Value
Total Fat 15g	23%
Saturated Fat 4.5g	23%
Trans Fat 0g	
Cholesterol 70mg	23%
Sodium 75mg	3%
Total Carbohydrate 9g	3%
Dietary Fiber 0g	0%
Sugars 9g	
Protein 28g	

Cold water fish, such as salmon, is an excellent source of Omega-3 fatty acids which are a heart healthy fat.

ORANGE-BASIL SALMON WITH GREEN BEANS

Number of Servings: 4

2 tsp	Orange zest, grated	**1 1/2 lbs**	Wild Alaskan salmon fillets
1/2 c	Orange juice		
1 Tbs	Fresh basil, chopped	**3/4 lb**	Green beans
1 Tbs	Fresh dill weed	**1 tsp**	Extra virgin olive oil
1 Tbs	Fresh ginger root	**1 tsp**	Minced garlic
1 tsp	Salt substitute	**1/4 tsp**	Salt substitute
1/2 tsp	Ground black pepper	**1/4 tsp**	Ground black pepper
1 tsp	Minced garlic		

Preheat oven to 450°. Position oven rack in top third of oven. Line baking pan with aluminum foil and coat with cooking spray. For the marinade, in a large shallow dish, whisk together orange zest, orange juice, basil, dill, ginger root, 1 teaspoon salt substitute, 1/2 teaspoon pepper and 1/2 teaspoon garlic. Reserve 2 tablespoons for later. Add salmon to dish and let sit for 15-20 minutes, turning fish occasionally. Transfer salmon to prepared pan, skin down. Roast 10-12 minutes.

To prepare the beans, bring a large saucepan of water to a boil. Add green beans and cook for about 10-12 minutes or until crisp-tender. Drain beans and toss with olive oil, 1 teaspoon garlic and 1/4 teaspoon each salt substitute and pepper. Transfer salmon and green beans to 4 plates and spoon reserved marinade over salmon.

Nutrition Facts

Serving Size 5-6 ounce fillet (295g)
Servings Per Container 4

Amount Per Serving

Calories 370 Calories from Fat 170

	% Daily Value
Total Fat 19g	29%
Saturated Fat 5g	25%
Trans Fat 0g	
Cholesterol 85mg	28%
Sodium 85mg	4%
Total Carbohydrate 11g	4%
Dietary Fiber 3g	12%
Sugars 4g	
Protein 36g	

 Submitted by Kate Brophy

THAI SALMON STEAKS

Number of Servings: 2

1 tsp	Rice vinegar		**2 Tbs**	Chinese mustard
2 Tbs	Low sodium soy sauce		**2 Tbs**	Fresh parsley, chopped
1/4 c	Light honey		**10 oz**	Pacific salmon fillets

Preheat grill. In a small sauce pan, combine the vinegar, soy sauce, honey, mustard and parsley. Simmer for about 5 minutes. Place steaks on the grill and cover each with a tablespoon of the Thai sauce. Close the grill and cook for 6 minutes. Check on salmon and continue grilling if needed. Serve with any remaining sauce.

Nutrition Facts

Serving Size 5 ounce fillet (222g)
Servings Per Container 2

Amount Per Serving

Calories 340 Calories from Fat 80

	% Daily Value
Total Fat 9g	14%
Saturated Fat 1.5g	8%
Trans Fat 0g	
Cholesterol 80mg	27%
Sodium 600mg	25%
Total Carbohydrate 36g	12%
Dietary Fiber 0g	0%
Sugars 32g	
Protein 29g	

MARK'S PECAN CRUSTED SALMON

Number of Servings: 4

4	5 oz wild Pacific salmon fillets	**1/4 c**	Plain whole wheat bread crumbs
4 tsp	Honey	**1/2 c**	Pecans, chopped
4 tsp	Dijon mustard	**2 tsp**	Fresh parsley, chopped
1/4 c	Plain bread crumbs		

Preheat oven to 450°. In a small bowl, combine honey with mustard and mix well; brush over salmon. In a small bowl, combine bread crumbs, pecans and parsley. Then spoon evenly across top of salmon. Bake for 12-15 minutes or until fish flakes easily with a fork. (Optional: Works well with grouper or other white fillets)

Nutrition Facts

Serving Size 5 ounce fillet (183g)
Servings Per Container 4

Amount Per Serving

Calories 380 Calories from Fat 180

	% Daily Value
Total Fat 20g	31%
Saturated Fat 2.5g	13%
Trans Fat 0g	
Cholesterol 80mg	27%
Sodium 230mg	10%
Total Carbohydrate 17g	6%
Dietary Fiber 2g	8%
Sugars 7g	
Protein 31g	

Submitted by Mark Hoesten

Keep a record of your exercise activities. Reward yourself at special milestones. Nothing motivates like success!

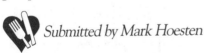

GROUPER CUTLETS WITH BLACK BEANS AND RELISH

Number of Servings: 4

1 1/2 lb	Grouper fillets	**1 Tbs**	Shallots, diced
1 1/2 c	Dry black beans	**1 tsp**	Extra virgin olive oil
1 Tbs	Extra virgin olive oil	**1 tsp**	Fresh cilantro, chopped
2 Tbs	All purpose flour	**1**	Fresh jalapeno pepper, seeded and diced
1/2 c	Fresh red tomatoes, peeled and seeded, chopped	**1 tsp**	Raspberry vinegar
		1/4 tsp	Ground black pepper
1 Tbs	Fresh ginger, finely diced	**1/4 tsp**	Salt substitute

Prepare relish in a small bowl by combining tomatoes, ginger, shallots, oil, cilantro, 1/2 jalapeno pepper, raspberry vinegar, pepper and salt substitute. Mix well and set aside.

Prepare grouper cutlets by pounding lightly with a mallet to flatten or use thinner fish fillets; cut into 2 oz slices. Season grouper with salt substitute and pepper, as desired. Heat 1 tablespoon olive oil in a large nonstick skillet over medium heat. Lightly flour grouper cutlets and quickly sauté in hot oil about 2-3 minutes on each side.

Cook beans as according to directions. Place grouper over warm black beans and spoon relish on top.

Nutrition Facts

Serving Size 5 ounce fillet and 1/3 cup black beans (281g)
Servings Per Container 4

Amount Per Serving

Calories 460   Calories from Fat 60

	% Daily Value
Total Fat 6g	9%
Saturated Fat 1g	5%
Trans Fat 0g	
Cholesterol 65mg	22%
Sodium 90mg	4%
Total Carbohydrate 49g	16%
Dietary Fiber 6g	24%
Sugars 7g	
Protein 48g	

CRAB CAKES

Number of Servings: 4

10 oz	Crab meat	**3 Tbs**	Fresh scallions, tops and bulbs, chopped
1	Omega-3 egg	**1/2 tsp**	Hot pepper sauce
3 Tbs	Fat free mayonnaise	**1/4 tsp**	Crab cake seasoning
1 Tbs	Dijon mustard	**2 tsp**	Canola oil
1/3 c	Plain bread crumbs		

Mix the crab, egg, mayonnaise, mustard, 1/4 cup of the bread crumbs, scallions, hot pepper sauce and crab seasoning in a large bowl. Form the mixture into four crab cakes. Place the remaining bread crumbs on a plate. Dredge both sides of the crab cakes into the bread crumbs to coat lightly. Place the crab cakes on a plate and set in the refrigerator for 30 minutes for the crab cakes to set. Heat the oil in a large nonstick skillet over medium-high heat. Add the crab cakes and sauté on both sides until golden brown, about 4-5 minutes per side.

Nutrition Facts

Serving Size 3 ounce crab cake (116g)
Servings Per Container 4

Amount Per Serving

Calories 150 Calories from Fat 45

	% Daily Value
Total Fat 5g	8%
Saturated Fat 0g	0%
Trans Fat 0g	
Cholesterol 95mg	32%
Sodium 480mg	20%
Total Carbohydrate 8g	3%
Dietary Fiber 1g	4%
Sugars 1g	
Protein 18g	

OVEN FRIED FISH

Number of Servings: 6

2 lbs	Cod fillets	**1/4 tsp**	Salt substitute
1 Tbs	Fresh lemon juice	**1/4 tsp**	Onion powder
1/4 c	Skim milk	**1/2 c**	Bread crumbs
1/8 tsp	Hot pepper sauce	**1 Tbs**	Canola oil
1 tsp	Minced garlic	**1**	Medium lemon
1/4 tsp	White pepper		

Preheat oven to 475°. Wipe fillets with lemon juice and pat dry. Combine milk, hot pepper sauce and garlic. Combine pepper, salt and onion powder with bread crumbs and place on a plate. Let fillets sit in milk mixture for 30 seconds. Remove and coat fillets on both sides with bread crumbs. Let stand briefly until coating sticks to each side of fish. Arrange on lightly oiled shallow baking dish. Bake 20 minutes on middle rack without turning. Cut into 6 pieces. Serve with fresh lemon wedges.

Nutrition Facts

Serving Size 5 ounce fillet (186g)
Servings Per Container 6

Amount Per Serving

Calories 190   Calories from Fat 35

	% Daily Value
Total Fat 4g	6%
Saturated Fat 0g	0%
Trans Fat 0g	
Cholesterol 55mg	18%
Sodium 180mg	8%
Total Carbohydrate 8g	3%
Dietary Fiber 1g	4%
Sugars 1g	
Protein 29g	

Activities that involve several of your larger muscles expend more energy. Skiing, football and tennis, for example, use larger muscles in your upper as well as lower body.

SHRIMP PASTA

Number of Servings: 6

1 lb	Medium shrimp	**4 oz**	Light cream cheese
1/2 c	Balsamic vinegar salad dressing	**3/4 lb**	Whole wheat fettuccini
2 c	Tomatoes, chopped	**1/4 c**	Reduced fat parmesan cheese, grated
1/2 c	Fresh basil leaves, chopped		

In a small bowl, pour dressing over shrimp; refrigerate 20 minutes to marinate. Remove shrimp from marinade; discard marinade.

Heat large skillet on medium heat; add shrimp. Cook 3 minutes or until shrimp turns pink, stirring frequently. Remove from skillet using slotted spoon; cover to keep warm. Set aside. Add tomatoes and half of the basil to same skillet; cook and stir 3 minutes. Stir in cream cheese until well blended. Add shrimp; cook until heated through, stirring occasionally.

Prepare fettuccini according to box directions. Place hot fettuccini on large serving platter. Top with the shrimp sauce. Sprinkle with remaining basil and the shredded cheese.

Nutrition Facts

Serving Size 3/4 cup (242g)
Servings Per Container 6

Amount Per Serving

Calories 380 Calories from Fat 110

	% Daily Value
Total Fat 12g	18%
Saturated Fat 2g	10%
Trans Fat 0g	
Cholesterol 130mg	43%
Sodium 580mg	24%
Total Carbohydrate 53g	18%
Dietary Fiber 8g	32%
Sugars 8g	
Protein 28g	

GRILLED TERIYAKI CHICKEN

Number of Servings: 4

1/3 c	Water	**2 tsp**	Minced garlic
1/8 c	Fat free reduced sodium chicken broth	**1/2 tsp**	Ground ginger
1/8 c	Low sodium soy sauce	**12 oz**	Boneless skinless chicken breasts

In a small saucepan, combine the first five ingredients. Bring to a boil over medium heat; cook for 1 minute. Cool for 10 minutes. Pour into re-sealable plastic bag; add chicken. Seal bag and turn to coat; refrigerate for at least 2 hours.

Drain and discard marinade. Grill chicken, covered, over medium heat for 7-8 minutes on each side or until juices run clear.

Nutrition Facts

Serving Size 3 ounce breast (122g)
Servings Per Container 4

Amount Per Serving	
Calories 110	Calories from Fat 10

	% Daily Value
Total Fat 1.5g	2%
Saturated Fat 0g	0%
Trans Fat 0g	
Cholesterol 50mg	17%
Sodium 340mg	14%
Total Carbohydrate 1g	0%
Dietary Fiber 0g	0%
Sugars 0g	
Protein 20g	

It is against the law to eat chicken with a fork in Gainesville, Georgia, the "Chicken Capital of the World."

THREE CHEESE CHICKEN PENNE FLORENTINE

Number of Servings: 8

1 tsp	Extra virgin olive oil	**1 lb**	Chicken breast strips, cooked
3 c	Mushrooms, sliced		
1 c	White onion, chopped	**1 c**	2% reduced fat sharp cheddar cheese, shredded
1 c	Red bell pepper, chopped		
3 c	Fresh spinach, chopped	**1/2 c**	Parmesan cheese, grated
1 Tbs	Oregano	**1/2 c**	1% milk
1/4 tsp	Ground black pepper	**1**	10 3/4 oz can 98% fat free 30% reduced sodium cream of chicken soup
16 oz	1% fat cottage cheese		
8 oz	Whole wheat penne pasta		

Preheat oven to 425°. Heat olive oil in a large nonstick skillet over medium-high heat. Add mushrooms, onion and bell pepper; sauté 4 minutes or until tender. Add spinach, oregano and black pepper; sauté 3 minutes or just until spinach wilts.

Place cottage cheese in food processor or blender; process until very smooth. Combine spinach mixture, cottage cheese, pasta, chicken, 3/4 cup cheddar cheese, 1/4 cup parmesan cheese, milk and undiluted soup in a large bowl. Spoon mixture into a 2-qt baking dish coated with nonstick cooking spray. Sprinkle with remaining 1/4 cup cheddar cheese and remaining 1/4 cup parmesan cheese. Bake for 25 minutes or until lightly browned and bubbly.

Nutrition Facts

Serving Size 1 cup (292g)
Servings Per Container 8

Amount Per Serving

Calories 330   Calories from Fat 80

	% Daily Value
Total Fat 9g	14%
Saturated Fat 3.5g	18%
Trans Fat 0g	
Cholesterol 50mg	17%
Sodium 850mg	35%
Total Carbohydrate 33g	11%
Dietary Fiber 4g	16%
Sugars 6g	
Protein 31g	

FETTUCCINI CACCIATORE

Number of Servings: 8

8 oz	Whole wheat fettuccini pasta	**1**	14 oz can no salt added diced tomatoes
2 tsp	Extra virgin olive oil	**1/4 c**	Fat free Italian salad dressing
1 lb	Skinless boneless chicken breasts, cubed	**1/2 c**	Mozzarella & parmesan cheese, finely shredded
1 c	Green bell pepper, sliced	**1/2 c**	Fresh basil, chopped
1 c	Fresh mushrooms, sliced		

Cook pasta as directed on package. Meanwhile, heat oil in large skillet on medium-high heat. Add chicken; cook and stir until no longer pink. Add peppers and mushrooms; cook 3 minutes, stirring occasionally. Stir in tomatoes with their liquid and the dressing. Reduce heat to medium-low; simmer 5 minutes or until chicken is cooked through. Toss pasta with chicken mixture. Sprinkle with cheese and basil.

Nutrition Facts

Serving Size 1 cup (163g)
Servings Per Container 8

Amount Per Serving	
Calories 200	Calories from Fat 60

	% Daily Value
Total Fat 6g	9%
Saturated Fat 1.5g	8%
Trans Fat 0g	
Cholesterol 30mg	10%
Sodium 190mg	8%
Total Carbohydrate 24g	8%
Dietary Fiber 4g	16%
Sugars 2g	
Protein 17g	

CHICKEN CORDON BLEU

Number of Servings: 12

1/4 c	Fat free low sodium chicken broth	**1 lb**	Boneless skinless chicken breasts
2 tsp	Trans fat free margarine	**1/4 tsp**	Salt substitute
1	Clove garlic, minced	**1/4 tsp**	Ground oregano
1/3 c	Plain bread crumbs	**1/4 tsp**	Ground black pepper
1 Tbs	Parmesan and romano cheese, grated	**1 oz**	Prosciutto, sliced
1 tsp	Paprika	**1/4 c**	Fat free mozzarella cheese, shredded

Place broth in a small microwave-safe bowl; microwave at HIGH 15 seconds or until warm. Stir in margarine and garlic. In a medium bowl, combine bread crumbs, parmesan and romano cheeses and paprika; set aside. Cut chicken breasts into halves. Place each breast half between two sheets of heavy duty plastic wrap and pound each to 1/4-inch thickness using a meat mallet or rolling pin.

Sprinkle both sides of chicken with salt substitute, oregano and pepper. Top each breast half with 1 slice of prosciutto (sliced very thin; you should be able to see through it) and 1 tablespoon mozzarella. Roll up each breast half, jellyroll fashion. Dip each roll in chicken broth mixture; dredge in bread crumb mixture. Place rolls, seam side down, into an 8-inch square baking dish coated with cooking spray. Pour remaining broth mixture over chicken and bake 28 minutes or until juices run clear.

Nutrition Facts

Serving Size 3 ounce (64g)
Servings Per Container 12

Amount Per Serving

Calories 150   Calories from Fat 60

% Daily Value

Total Fat 6g	9%
Saturated Fat 1.5g	8%
Trans Fat 0g	
Cholesterol 30mg	10%
Sodium 520mg	22%
Total Carbohydrate 12g	4%
Dietary Fiber 0g	0%
Sugars 0g	
Protein 12g	

TURKEY BURGERS WITH SAUCE

Number of Servings: 2

1/4 c	Red onion, chopped	**1 tsp**	Dried chives
2 Tbs	Parsley, dried	**1 1/2 tsp**	Fresh basil, finely chopped
1 Tbs	Light sour cream		
1/3 c	Light sour cream	**1 1/2 tsp**	Lemon juice
8 oz	99% fat free ground turkey	**3/4 tsp**	Tarragon
		1/8 tsp	Salt substitute
1 Tbs	Reduced fat feta cheese	**1/8 tsp**	Ground black pepper

Combine onion, parsley and 1 tablespoon of light sour cream. Crumble turkey over mixture and mix well. Make 4 patties. Top 2 of the patties with feta cheese and with remaining turkey mixture press on top of first 2 patties (a feta cheese stuffed burger). Grill over medium-high heat or broil 4-6 inches from heat for 5-6 minutes on each side.

Nutrition Facts

Serving Size 3 ounce burger (197g)
Servings Per Container 2

Amount Per Serving	
Calories 200 Calories from Fat 50	
	% Daily Value
Total Fat 5g	8%
Saturated Fat 3g	15%
Trans Fat 0g	
Cholesterol 65mg	22%
Sodium 310mg	13%
Total Carbohydrate 10g	3%
Dietary Fiber 1g	4%
Sugars 4g	
Protein 31g	

In a smaller bowl, combine chives, basil, lemon juice, tarragon, salt, pepper and rest of sour cream. Serve patties with herb sauce.

FETTUCCINI ALFREDO

Number of Servings: 4

8 oz Whole wheat fettuccini pasta
1 1/4 c Fat free reduced sodium chicken broth
4 tsp All purpose flour
1/3 c Soft light cream cheese

3 Tbs Parmesan cheese, grated
1/8 tsp Ground nutmeg
2 Tbs Fresh parsley, chopped

Cook pasta as directed on package. Meanwhile, combine broth and flour in medium saucepan. Stir in cream cheese; cook several minutes, stirring constantly until mixture boils and thickens. Toss pasta with sauce, 2 tablespoons of parmesan cheese and the nutmeg. Sprinkle with remaining 1 tablespoon parmesan cheese and the parsley. Season to taste with pepper.

Nutrition Facts

Serving Size 1 cup (150g)
Servings Per Container 4

Amount Per Serving

Calories 280   Calories from Fat 50

	% Daily Value
Total Fat 5g	8%
Saturated Fat 3g	15%
Trans Fat 0g	
Cholesterol 15mg	5%
Sodium 300mg	13%
Total Carbohydrate 44g	15%
Dietary Fiber 1g	4%
Sugars 3g	
Protein 11g	

When reading the ingredient list on the food label, the flour used should be preceded by the word "whole," such as "whole wheat flour" or "whole rye flour," etc.

MEATLOAF

Number of Servings: 8

2 lbs	99% fat free ground turkey breast	**1**	Omega-3 egg
1 lb	96% lean ground beef	**2 tsp**	Worcestershire sauce
1	Yellow onion, chopped	**1/2 c**	Bread crumbs
1/4 c	Parmesan & romano cheese, grated	**1/2 c**	Skim milk
		2 c	No salt added tomato sauce

Preheat oven to 350°. Mix together all ingredients. Put into meatloaf pan that drains any grease. Bake for approximately one hour. (Optional: spread tomato sauce over the top). Let cool 15 minutes before serving.

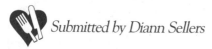 *Submitted by Diann Sellers*

Nutrition Facts

Serving Size 1-inch slice (309g)
Servings Per Container 8

Amount Per Serving	
Calories 310 Calories from Fat 80	
	% Daily Value
Total Fat 8g	12%
Saturated Fat 2.5g	13%
Trans Fat 0g	
Cholesterol 205mg	68%
Sodium 280mg	12%
Total Carbohydrate 13g	4%
Dietary Fiber 1g	4%
Sugars 2g	
Protein 47g	

For the first 20 minutes you exercise in your aerobic zone, you are burning about 80% carbohydrates and 20% fat. For the next 20 minutes, you are burning 50% carbs and 50% fat. If you start exercising into the above 40 minute range, you are now burning about 20% carbs and about 80% fat.

GREEN BEAN JULIENNE

Number of Servings: 8

16 oz	Frozen French cut green beans	**1 Tbs**	Apple cider vinegar
1/2 c	Red bell peppers, sliced	**1 tsp**	Sesame oil
1 tsp	Extra virgin olive oil	**2 tsp**	Ground ginger
2 Tbs	Shallots, chopped	**1 tsp**	Chinese five spice blend
1 Tbs	Low sodium soy sauce	**1 Tbs**	Sesame seeds

In a large saucepan, sauté the minced shallots in the soy sauce, olive oil, sesame oil, ground ginger and five spice powder until shallots are softened. Add the red pepper strips and continue to cook over medium-high heat for 3 minutes. Add the thawed green beans and continue cooking until the beans have been heated through and are coated with the sauce and shallots. Add sesame seeds and serve.

Nutrition Facts

Serving Size 1/2 cup (72g)
Servings Per Container 8

Amount Per Serving

Calories 40   Calories from Fat 15

	% Daily Value
Total Fat 2g	3%
Saturated Fat 0g	0%
Trans Fat 0g	
Cholesterol 0mg	0%
Sodium 70mg	3%
Total Carbohydrate 6g	2%
Dietary Fiber 2g	8%
Sugars 2g	
Protein 1g	

GREENS

Number of Servings: 5

3 c	Water	**2 tsp**	Minced garlic
4 oz	Roasted skinless boneless turkey breast, cooked, diced	**1/2 tsp**	Ground thyme
		2 Tbs	Scallions, tops and bulbs, chopped
1 Tbs	Fresh red hot chili peppers, chopped	**1 tsp**	Ground ginger
		1/4 c	White onion, chopped
1/4 tsp	Ground cayenne pepper	**2 lb**	Mustard greens, chopped
1/4 tsp	Ground cloves		

Place all ingredients except greens into large saucepan and bring to a boil. Prepare greens by washing thoroughly and removing stems. Chop greens and add them to the turkey stock. You can mix mustard, turnip, collard or kale greens if desired. Cook 20-30 minutes until tender.

Nutrition Facts

Serving Size 1 cup (356g)
Servings Per Container 5

Amount Per Serving	
Calories 80	Calories from Fat 5

	% Daily Value
Total Fat 1g	2%
Saturated Fat 0g	0%
Trans Fat 0g	
Cholesterol 15mg	5%
Sodium 60mg	3%
Total Carbohydrate 11g	4%
Dietary Fiber 6g	24%
Sugars 3g	
Protein 11g	

STUFFED PORTABELLA MUSHROOMS

Number of Servings: 4

3	Portabella mushrooms	**2 oz**	Low fat Swiss cheese, shredded
1/4 c	Yellow onion, chopped	**3 oz**	2% reduced fat monterey jack cheese
1 1/2 Tbs	Garlic, crushed	**1/4 c**	Almonds, sliced
9 oz	Fresh baby spinach		

Preheat oven to 350°. Clean mushrooms and scrape out insides. Pre-cook for about 10 minutes by placing the mushrooms upside down on a cookie sheet. Meanwhile, sauté onions and garlic. Add spinach and cover with lid until spinach cooks down. Add the cheeses and almonds. Fill mushrooms with mixture and bake for about 10-15 minutes.

Nutrition Facts

Serving Size 1/2 mushroom (184g)
Servings Per Container 4

Amount Per Serving	
Calories 190 Calories from Fat 80	
	% Daily Value
Total Fat 9g	14%
Saturated Fat 3.5g	18%
Trans Fat 0g	
Cholesterol 20mg	7%
Sodium 320mg	13%
Total Carbohydrate 13g	4%
Dietary Fiber 5g	20%
Sugars 2g	
Protein 14g	

JULIE'S SWEET POTATO CRUNCH

Number of Servings: 6

3	5-inch long sweet potatoes, peeled, boiled, mashed	**1 tsp**	Vanilla extract
		2	Omega-3 eggs
3/4 c	Splenda®	**1/4 c**	Splenda® brown sugar blend
1/2 c	Skim milk	**2 1/2 Tbs**	Trans fat free margarine
1 Tbs	Trans fat free margarine	**1/3 c**	Whole wheat flour
1/2 tsp	Salt substitute	**1/3 c**	Walnuts, chopped

Preheat oven to 350°. In a large bowl, combine the first 7 ingredients; mix well and put into greased 8x8-inch dish. Mix remaining ingredients for topping and cover top of potato mixture. Bake for 45 minutes.

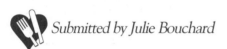 *Submitted by Julie Bouchard*

Nutrition Facts

Serving Size 1/2 cup (136g)
Servings Per Container 6

Amount Per Serving	
Calories 270 Calories from Fat 110	
	% Daily Value
Total Fat 12g	18%
Saturated Fat 2g	10%
Trans Fat 0g	
Cholesterol 60mg	20%
Sodium 135mg	6%
Total Carbohydrate 23g	8%
Dietary Fiber 3g	12%
Sugars 12g	
Protein 6g	

ROASTED CARROTS & ONIONS WITH WILD MUSHROOMS

Number of Servings: 8

1 1/2 lb	Pearl onions		**3 oz**	Oyster mushrooms, sliced
1 lb	Baby carrots			
16	Twigs fresh thyme		**3 oz**	Shitake mushrooms, discard stems
2 Tbs	Extra virgin olive oil			
1 1/2 tsp	Ground black pepper		**2 Tbs**	Light unsalted butter
			1/2 c	Fat free reduced sodium chicken broth
3 oz	Crimini mushrooms, quartered		**2 Tbs**	Balsamic vinegar

Preheat oven to 450°. Bring a large pot of water to a boil. Add onions and cook for 2 minutes, then drain and cool. Trim the stem and root ends and slip off the skins. (If using frozen pearl onions, skip this step and defrost according to package directions). Spread onions and carrots on two rimmed baking sheets. Add the thyme, olive oil and 1/4 teaspoon pepper to each tray. Toss until vegetables are lightly coated. Roast about 25 minutes, stirring several times, until lightly caramelized and slightly tender. Cool and discard the thyme sprigs.

Melt butter in a large skillet over medium high heat. Combine mushrooms and sauté until tender, about 4-6 minutes. Add carrots, onions, broth and vinegar. Cook, tossing until heated through, about 3-4 minutes. Add remaining 1/4 teaspoon of pepper and serve.

Nutrition Facts

Serving Size 2/3 cup (199g)
Servings Per Container 8

Amount Per Serving

Calories 130   Calories from Fat 45

	% Daily Value
Total Fat 5g	8%
Saturated Fat 1.5g	8%
Trans Fat 0g	
Cholesterol 5mg	2%
Sodium 65mg	3%
Total Carbohydrate 18g	6%
Dietary Fiber 3g	12%
Sugars 8g	
Protein 3g	

GLAZED CARROTS

Number of Servings: 8

4 c	Fresh carrots, sliced	**1 Tbs**	Low sodium Worcestershire sauce
1/2 c	Fat free Catalina salad dressing	**2 Tbs**	Fresh parsley, chopped
2 Tbs	Brown sugar		

In a medium saucepan, cook carrots in boiling water until crisp-tender; drain. Return to saucepan. Add dressing, brown sugar and Worcestershire sauce; stir until evenly coated. Cook on low heat for 5 minutes or until brown sugar is completely melted and carrots are evenly coated with the glaze, stirring frequently. Stir in parsley.

Nutrition Facts

Serving Size 1/2 cup (84g)
Servings Per Container 8

Amount Per Serving

Calories 50   Calories from Fat 0

	% Daily Value
Total Fat 0g	0%
Saturated Fat 0g	0%
Trans Fat 0g	
Cholesterol 0mg	0%
Sodium 210mg	9%
Total Carbohydrate 13g	4%
Dietary Fiber 2g	8%
Sugars 9g	
Protein 1g	

Large or older carrots can have a slightly bitter taste. To store carrots, cut the tops off and place them in a plastic bag in the vegetable crisper. Avoid carrots with green tops; they will be bitter.

INDIAN POTATOES

Number of Servings: 6

6	Red potatoes (not russet)	**1 Tbs**	Fresh cilantro, chopped
1 tsp	Ground cumin	**1 1/2 Tbs**	Canola oil
1 tsp	Ground tumeric	**1 tsp**	Salt substitute

Boil the potatoes so they are firm but done. Slice each potato into 8 wedges. Heat oil in a large skillet over medium heat. Add cumin and tumeric to the hot oil and mix quickly. Add the potatoes and cilantro. Mix well and sauté briefly. Add salt substitute to taste and remove from heat. Serve hot.

Nutrition Facts

Serving Size 1/2 cup (153g)
Servings Per Container 6

Amount Per Serving

Calories 70   Calories from Fat 30

% Daily Value

Total Fat 3.5g	5%
Saturated Fat 0g	0%
Trans Fat 0g	
Cholesterol 0mg	0%
Sodium 10mg	0%
Total Carbohydrate 7g	2%
Dietary Fiber 4g	16%
Sugars 2g	
Protein 3g	

WILD RICE PILAF

Number of Servings: 8

1/2 c	White onion, chopped	**4 oz**	Dried apricots
2 tsp	Canola oil	**2 Tbs**	Fresh parsley, chopped
6 oz	Brown rice, cooked	**2 Tbs**	Fresh orange juice
1 1/3 c	Fat free reduced sodium chicken broth	**2 tsp**	Balsamic vinegar
1/2 c	Frozen green peas, thawed and drained	**1/2 tsp**	Salt substitute
1	Green onion, top and bulb, chopped	**1/8 tsp**	Ground black pepper

In a saucepan, sauté chopped onion in oil until tender. Add rice (a brown rice/wild rice mix can be substituted) and broth; bring to a boil. Reduce heat; cover and simmer 25-30 minutes or until liquid is absorbed. Remove from heat; stir in the remaining ingredients. Cover and let stand for 5 minutes.

Nutrition Facts

Serving Size 1/2 cup (99g)

Servings Per Container 8

Amount Per Serving

Calories 90   Calories from Fat 10

% Daily Value

Total Fat 1.5g	2%
Saturated Fat 0g	0%
Trans Fat 0g	
Cholesterol 0mg	0%
Sodium 85mg	4%
Total Carbohydrate 17g	6%
Dietary Fiber 2g	8%
Sugars 1g	
Protein 2g	

Strength training exercises use resistance – for example, weights or bodyweight—to condition the musculoskeletal system, improving muscle tone and endurance.

HARVEST MUFFINS

Number of Servings: 12

1/2 c	Water	1/2 c	Unsweetened applesauce
3/4 tsp	Cream of tartar	1/2 c	Pureed carrots (baby food)
1 1/4 c	Old fashioned oats	1 c	Fresh carrots, grated
1 3/4 c	Oat flour	3 oz	Unsweetened apple juice
3/4 tsp	Baking soda	1/2 c	Walnuts, chopped
1/8 tsp	Ground nutmeg	3	Egg whites
1/3 c	Honey		
1 1/2 tsp	Ground cinnamon		
2 tsp	Vanilla extract		

Preheat oven to 350°. In a large bowl, combine oats with oat flour, baking soda, cream of tartar, cinnamon and nutmeg; mix well. Set aside.

In a medium bowl, mix together honey, vanilla, applesauce, carrot puree, grated carrots, orange juice concentrate and water; pour into oat mixture. Stir to blend. Stir in nuts. Gently mix in lightly beaten egg whites. Do not over mix.

Pour into muffin pan which has been sprayed with nonstick cooking spray. Bake for 25 minutes or until toothpick inserted in center comes out clean. Cool on a wire rack for 10 minutes and remove muffins from pan.

Nutrition Facts

Serving Size 1 muffin (176g)
Servings Per Container 12

Amount Per Serving

Calories 400   Calories from Fat 60

	% Daily Value
Total Fat 7g	11%
Saturated Fat 1g	5%
Trans Fat 0g	
Cholesterol 0mg	0%
Sodium 200mg	8%
Total Carbohydrate 55g	18%
Dietary Fiber 7g	28%
Sugars 12g	
Protein 15g	

SAVORY ADD-A-CRUNCH

Number of Servings: 24

2 c Dry old fashioned oats
1/2 c Trans fat free margarine
1/3 c Parmesan cheese, grated

1/3 c Wheat germ, toasted
1/4 tsp Garlic salt

Preheat oven to 350°. Combine all ingredients; mix well. Bake in ungreased 15 1/2x10 1/2-inch jelly roll pan for 15-18 minutes or until light golden brown. Cool; store in tightly covered container in refrigerator up to 3 months. Sprinkle over tossed green salads, soups, casseroles or vegetables.

Variation: add 1 teaspoon oregano leaves and 1/2 teaspoon thyme leaves to mixture before baking.

Microwave oven directions: Cook in ungreased 11x7-inch baking dish on HIGH for 8-9 minutes or our until light golden brown, stirring after every 3 minutes of cooking. Cool.

Nutrition Facts	
Serving Size 2 tablespoons (14g)	
Servings Per Container 24	
Amount Per Serving	
Calories 70 Calories from Fat 40	
	% Daily Value
Total Fat 4.5g	7%
Saturated Fat 0.5g	3%
Trans Fat 0g	
Cholesterol 0mg	0%
Sodium 55mg	2%
Total Carbohydrate 5g	2%
Dietary Fiber 1g	4%
Sugars 0g	
Protein 2g	

CORN MUFFINS

Number of Servings: 24

1 c	Whole grain cornmeal	**1**	Omega-3 egg
1/4 c	All purpose flour	**1 c**	Plain fat free yogurt
2 tsp	Baking powder	**1/2 c**	Skim milk
1/2 tsp	Salt substitute	**1/4 c**	Canola oil
1/4 tsp	Baking soda	**1 Tbs**	Honey

Preheat oven to 425°. In a large bowl, combine the first five ingredients. In another bowl, combine the egg, yogurt, milk, oil and honey. Then stir into dry ingredients just until moistened. Pour into mini or regular muffin cups or 8-inch square pan coated with nonstick cooking spray. Bake for 14-18 minutes or until a toothpick comes out clean. Makes 12 regular muffins, 24 mini muffins or 9 servings from square pan.

Nutrition Facts

Serving Size 1 mini muffin (27g)
Servings Per Container 24

Amount Per Serving

Calories 60   Calories from Fat 25

	% Daily Value
Total Fat 2.5g	4%
Saturated Fat 0g	0%
Trans Fat 0g	
Cholesterol 10mg	3%
Sodium 70mg	3%
Total Carbohydrate 7g	2%
Dietary Fiber 0g	0%
Sugars 2g	
Protein 1g	

TASSAJARA GRANOLA

Number of Servings: 24

4 1/2 c	Old fashioned oats	**1 Tbs**	Vanilla extract
3 c	Almonds, slivered	**1 1/2 tsp**	Ground cinnamon
1 1/2 c	Sunflower seeds	**1/2 tsp**	Almond extract
1 1/2 c	Dried pumpkin kernels and squash seeds	**1/8 tsp**	Ground clove
		3/4 c	Canola oil
1 1/4 c	Honey	**1 1/2 tsp**	Salt substitute
1/4 c	Maple syrup		

Preheat oven to 325°. Put the oats, slivered almonds and sunflower, pumpkin and squash seeds in a large bowl. In a small saucepan, combine the oil, honey, maple syrup, vanilla, almond extract, spices and salt. Heat the mixture over low heat until it becomes watery. Pour the oil mixture over the dry ingredients, tossing until everything is moistened. Spread the mixture in a large baking pan or cookie sheet. Bake in the middle of the oven for about 20 minutes, or until the granola turns golden, stirring every 5 minutes so the mixture toasts uniformly. Transfer to a large bowl or cool baking pan and toss occasionally until the granola is thoroughly cool and dry. Store in a tightly covered container.

Nutrition Facts

Serving Size 1/2 cup (63g)
Servings Per Container 24

Amount Per Serving

Calories 340 Calories from Fat 210

	% Daily Value
Total Fat 24g	37%
Saturated Fat 2.5g	13%
Trans Fat 0g	
Cholesterol 0mg	0%
Sodium 160mg	7%
Total Carbohydrate 24g	8%
Dietary Fiber 5g	20%
Sugars 6g	
Protein 10g	

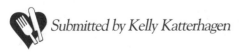

Submitted by Kelly Katterhagen

APPLE-PEANUT BUTTER CRISP

Number of Servings: 6

1/4 c	Whole wheat flour	**3 Tbs**	Natural peanut butter
1/2 c	Splenda®	**3 Tbs**	Trans fat free
1/2 tsp	Salt substitute		margarine
1/4 c	Old fashioned oats	**5 c**	Apples, peeled, sliced

Preheat oven to 350°. In a small mixing bowl, stir together flour, Splenda® and salt substitute. Cut in peanut butter and margarine until mixture resembles coarse crumbs. Place sliced apples in a greased 12x7-inch baking dish. Sprinkle peanut butter mixture evenly over apples. Bake about 45 minutes or until apples are tender. Serve warm or cooled. If desired, serve with low fat no sugar added ice cream.

Nutrition Facts

Serving Size 1/2 cup (117g)
Servings Per Container 6

Amount Per Serving

Calories 170 Calories from Fat 80

	% Daily Value
Total Fat 9g	14%
Saturated Fat 2g	10%
Trans Fat 0g	
Cholesterol 0mg	0%
Sodium 85mg	4%
Total Carbohydrate 21g	7%
Dietary Fiber 3g	12%
Sugars 10g	
Protein 3g	

When purchasing fresh apples, look for firm, crisp, well-colored apples. Overripe apples (indicated by a yielding to slight pressure on the skin and soft, mealy flesh), apples affected by freeze (indicated by internal breakdown and bruised areas) and scald on apples (irregularly shaped tan or brown areas) may not seriously affect the taste.

ORANGE NUT WHOLE WHEAT CAKE

Number of Servings: 9

1 1/4 c All purpose flour
1 c Whole wheat flour
1/2 c Splenda® brown sugar blend
1 tsp Baking soda
1/2 tsp Salt substitute

1 c Orange juice
1/2 c Canola oil
1 tsp Orange peel, grated
1 Omega-3 egg
1/2 c Walnuts, chopped

Preheat oven to 350°. Grease and flour 8 or 9-inch square pan. In a large bowl, combine all ingredients except walnuts; beat for 2 minutes at medium speed. Stir in walnuts. Pour batter into prepared pan. Bake for 40-50 minutes or until toothpick inserted in center comes out clean.

Nutrition Facts

Serving Size 2-inch square (94g)
Servings Per Container 9

Amount Per Serving	
Calories 330 Calories from Fat 160	
	% Daily Value
Total Fat 18g	28%
Saturated Fat 1.5g	8%
Trans Fat 0g	
Cholesterol 20mg	7%
Sodium 140mg	6%
Total Carbohydrate 26g	9%
Dietary Fiber 2g	8%
Sugars 14g	
Protein 5g	

A whole grain kernel has three parts: the bran, the endosperm and the germ. Bran contains B vitamins, iron and fiber, the endosperm is mostly starch and some protein and the germ contains fatty acids and vitamin E.

CHOCOLATE OATMEAL BOILED COOKIES

Number of Servings: 42

2 c	Splenda®
1/2 c	Skim milk
1/2 c	Trans fat free margarine
3 Tbs	Cocoa powder, unsweetened

1/2 c	Natural peanut butter
3 c	Old fashioned oats
1 tsp	Vanilla extract

Put Splenda®, milk, margarine and cocoa powder in a large saucepan. Stir continuously and bring to boil for 1 minute. Remove from heat and beat in peanut butter, oats and vanilla. Drop by teaspoonful onto wax paper. Let stand until cool.

Nutrition Facts

Serving Size 1 tablespoon sized cookie (16g)
Servings Per Container 42

Amount Per Serving	
Calories 60	Calories from Fat 35

	% Daily Value
Total Fat 3.5g	5%
Saturated Fat 1g	5%
Trans Fat 0g	
Cholesterol 0mg	0%
Sodium 35mg	1%
Total Carbohydrate 6g	2%
Dietary Fiber 1g	4%
Sugars 1g	
Protein 2g	

MARCIA'S MARBLED CHOCOLATE BANANA BREAD

Number of Servings: 16

1 c	All purpose flour	**1 1/2 c**	Banana, mashed
1 c	Whole wheat flour	**1/2 c**	Egg substitute
3/4 tsp	Baking Soda	**1/3 c**	Plain nonfat yogurt
1/2 tsp	Salt substitute	**1/2 c**	Semi sweet
1/2 c	Sugar		chocolate chips
1/4 c	Trans fat free margarine		

Preheat oven to 350°. Lightly spoon flours into dry measuring cups; level with a knife. Combine flours, baking soda and salt substitute, stirring with a whisk. Place sugar and margarine in a large bowl; beat at medium speed until well blended (about 1 minute). Add banana, egg substitute and yogurt, beat until blended. Add the flour mixture, beat at low speed just until moist.

Nutrition Facts

Serving Size 1-inch slice (64g)
Servings Per Container 16

Amount Per Serving	
Calories 140 Calories from Fat 35	
	% Daily Value
Total Fat 4g	6%
Saturated Fat 1.5g	8%
Trans Fat 0g	
Cholesterol 0mg	0%
Sodium 100mg	4%
Total Carbohydrate 26g	9%
Dietary Fiber 1g	4%
Sugars 13g	
Protein 3g	

Place chocolate chips in a medium microwave safe bowl and microwave at HIGH 1 minute or until almost melted, stirring until smooth. Cool slightly. Add 1 cup batter to chocolate, stirring until well combined. Spoon chocolate batter alternately with plain batter into an 8 1/2 x 4 1/2-inch loaf pan coated with cooking spray. Swirl batters together using a knife. Bake for 1 hour and 15 minutes or until a wooden pick inserted in center comes out clean. Cool 10 minutes in pan on a wire rack; remove from pan. Cool completely on wire rack.

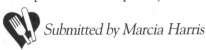 *Submitted by Marcia Harris*

CINNAMON ADD-A-CRUNCH

Number of Servings: 32

1 1/4 c Old fashioned oats
1/8 c Splenda®
1/8 c Brown sugar, packed
1/3 c Trans fat free
margarine

1/3 c Toasted wheat germ
1/4 tsp Ground cinnamon

In a medium bowl, combine all ingredients; mix well. Pour into a 10-inch skillet and cook over medium heat, stirring constantly, 5-7 minutes or until golden brown. Spread onto ungreased cookie sheet to cool. Store in tightly covered container in refrigerator up to 3 months. Serve as topping over fruit salad, fruit, yogurt, frozen yogurt, ice cream or pudding.

Nutrition Facts

Serving Size 1 tablespoon (8g)
Servings Per Container 32

Amount Per Serving	
Calories 35	Calories from Fat 20

	% Daily Value
Total Fat 2g	3%
Saturated Fat 0g	0%
Trans Fat 0g	
Cholesterol 0mg	0%
Sodium 15mg	1%
Total Carbohydrate 4g	1%
Dietary Fiber 0g	0%
Sugars 1g	
Protein 1g	

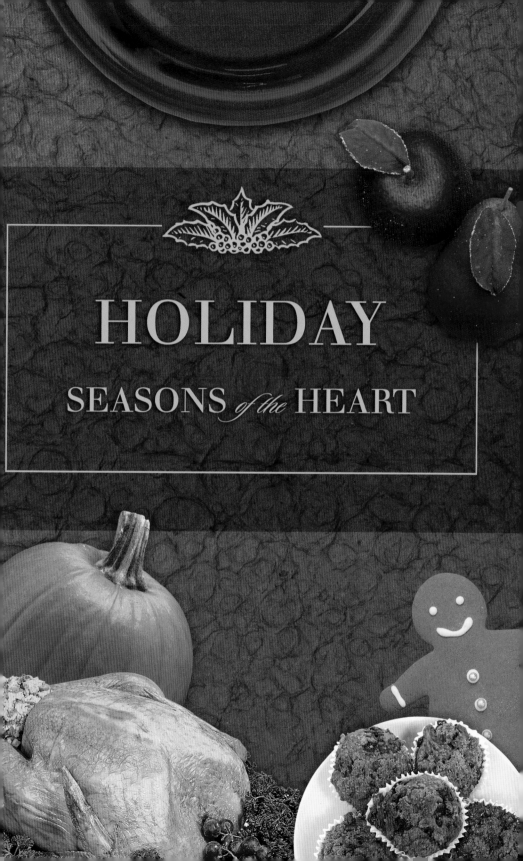

HOLIDAY

SEASONS *of the* HEART

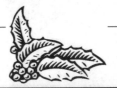

GINGER-CINNAMON FRUIT DIP

Number of Servings: 8

6 oz Low fat vanilla yogurt
1/4 c Low fat cream cheese, whipped

1 tsp Ground ginger
1/4 tsp Ground cinnamon

In a small bowl, combine yogurt, cream cheese, ginger and cinnamon until well blended. Chill at least 1 hour. Serve with fruit.

Nutrition Facts

Serving Size 2 tablespoons (27g)
Servings Per Container 8

Amount Per Serving

Calories 30   Calories from Fat 10

	% Daily Value
Total Fat 1g	2%
Saturated Fat 0.5g	3%
Trans Fat 0g	
Cholesterol 5mg	2%
Sodium 30mg	1%
Total Carbohydrate 4g	1%
Dietary Fiber 0g	0%
Sugars 3g	
Protein 2g	

If a recipe must have fat to work, try using half the fat called for. You will have to experiment, but in the majority of recipes, you can reduce the fat content to some degree.

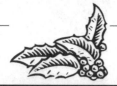

PARMESAN YOGURT DIP

Number of Servings: 10

1 c Plain nonfat yogurt
1/4 c Parmesan cheese, grated
1/4 c Light sour cream
3 Tbs Fresh parsley, chopped
1 Green onion, top and bulb, chopped

1 tsp Mustard
1 tsp Onion powder
1/4 tsp Salt substitute
1/8 tsp Ground black pepper

In a bowl, combine all ingredients. Cover and refrigerate for at least 2 hours. Serve with assorted vegetables.

Nutrition Facts

Serving Size 2 tablespoons (43g)
Servings Per Container 10

Amount Per Serving	
Calories 30	Calories from Fat 10

	% Daily Value
Total Fat 1g	2%
Saturated Fat 1g	5%
Trans Fat 0g	
Cholesterol 5mg	2%
Sodium 55mg	2%
Total Carbohydrate 3g	1%
Dietary Fiber 0g	0%
Sugars 2g	
Protein 2g	

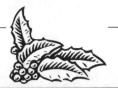

HOT CRAB DIP

Number of Servings: 24

8 oz Light cream cheese
8 oz Fat free cream cheese
12 oz Crab meat
1/4 c White onion, chopped
2 Tbs Horseradish sauce
2 tsp Worcestershire sauce
1/4 tsp Hot pepper sauce

1/4 c White wine
2 Tbs Whole wheat bread crumbs
5 Sprays of liquid spray margarine
1/8 tsp Ground paprika

Preheat oven to 350°. Coat the inside of 1 quart round baking dish with nonstick cooking spray. In a medium bowl, stir cream cheeses until smooth. Fold in crabmeat, onion, horseradish, Worcestershire sauce, hot sauce and wine. Spoon into baking dish. In a separate small bowl, toss bread crumbs, paprika and liquid margarine making sure to coat the crumbs completely. Spread bread crumb mixture evenly on top of crab dip mixture. Bake, uncovered, for 20 minutes or until bubbly and hot. Serve immediately with an assortment of whole grain crackers.

Nutrition Facts

Serving Size 2 tablespoons (40g)
Servings Per Container 24

Amount Per Serving

Calories 50 Calories from Fat 20

% Daily Value

Total Fat 2g	3%
Saturated Fat 1g	5%
Trans Fat 0g	
Cholesterol 15mg	5%
Sodium 170mg	7%
Total Carbohydrate 2g	1%
Dietary Fiber 0g	0%
Sugars 1g	
Protein 5g	

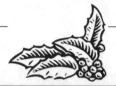

RICOTTA PESTO DIP

Number of Servings: 8

1 c	Fat free ricotta cheese	**1/2 tsp**	Fresh thyme, chopped
1/2 c	Sun dried tomatoes, diced	**1/2 Tbs**	Extra virgin olive oil
2	Garlic cloves, chopped	**1/8 tsp**	Ground black pepper
1	Roma tomato, chopped	**2 Tbs**	Shallots, diced
1/4 c	Fresh basil leaves, chopped	**3 oz**	Reduced fat feta cheese

Combine ricotta and feta cheeses. Blend completely. Cover and refrigerate. To make salsa, place the sun dried tomatoes in a heat proof bowl and add boiling water to cover. Let stand until softened and very pliable, 25-30 minutes. Drain. Squeeze dry and chop coarsely. In a separate bowl, make the pesto by combining the sun dried tomatoes, garlic, shallots, tomatoes, basil and thyme. Add the olive oil and pepper, and toss until well blended. Cover and refrigerate until serving.

To serve, mound the cheese on a serving platter. Put the pesto on the cheese. Spoon the salsa on and around the edge of the cheese mound. Garnish with fresh basil leaves. Serve with whole grain crackers.

Nutrition Facts

Serving Size 2 tablespoons (63g)
Servings Per Container 8

Amount Per Serving

Calories 70   Calories from Fat 20

	% Daily Value
Total Fat 2g	3%
Saturated Fat 1g	5%
Trans Fat 0g	
Cholesterol 10mg	3%
Sodium 240mg	10%
Total Carbohydrate 7g	2%
Dietary Fiber 1g	4%
Sugars 3g	
Protein 6g	

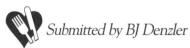

Submitted by BJ Denzler

WHITE BEAN AND WALNUT DIP

Number of Servings: 6

1 c	Mushrooms, chopped	**1 Tbs**	Parsley, minced
1/4 c	White onion, chopped	**1 Tbs**	Fresh basil, chopped
1 tsp	Minced garlic	**1Tbs**	Cooking wine
1	15 oz can of Navy beans, drained and rinsed	**2 tsp**	Worcestershire sauce
		1/4 tsp	Hot pepper sauce
1/2 c	Toasted walnuts, finely chopped		

Coat a large skillet with nonstick cooking spray. Place over medium heat until warm. Add mushrooms, onions and garlic. Cook for 10 minutes, or until most of the liquid has evaporated. Transfer to a food processor or blender. Add the beans, walnuts, parsley, basil, cooking wine and Worcestershire sauce. Process until smooth. Season with hot sauce. Add salt substitute and pepper to taste. Transfer to a medium bowl. Store tightly covered in the refrigerator for up to 2 days.

Nutrition Facts

Serving Size 1/4 cup (212g)
Servings Per Container 6

Amount Per Serving

Calories 160   Calories from Fat 60

	% Daily Value
Total Fat 7g	20%
Saturated Fat 0g	0%
Trans Fat 0g	
Cholesterol 0mg	0%
Sodium 360mg	15%
Total Carbohydrate 18g	6%
Dietary Fiber 5g	18%
Sugars 1g	
Protein 8g	

SPINACH DIP

Number of Servings: 12

1 10 oz box of frozen chopped spinach, thawed and drained

8 oz Fat free sour cream
1 Packet of powdered ranch dressing

In a large bowl, combine all ingredients, mix well and chill. Serve in hollowed whole grain bread with whole grain crackers or vegetables.

Nutrition Facts

Serving Size 2 tablespoons (44g)
Servings Per Container 12

Amount Per Serving

Calories 25   Calories from Fat 0

% Daily Value

Total Fat 0g	0%
Saturated Fat 0g	0%
Trans Fat 0g	
Cholesterol 0mg	0%
Sodium 115mg	5%
Total Carbohydrate 5g	2%
Dietary Fiber 1g	4%
Sugars 0g	
Protein 2g	

In most recipes, you can use fat free cream cheese or blended fat free cottage cheese instead of regular cream cheese. For recipes where fat content is necessary, try using half regular cream cheese and half reduced or fat free cream cheese.

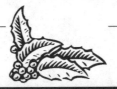

DOUBLE PEANUT
SNACK MIX

Number of Servings: 8

4 c Bite size shredded wheat cereal
1 c Unsalted dry roasted peanuts

1/4 c Trans fat free margarine
1/4 c Natural peanut butter
1 tsp Ground cinnamon

Preheat oven to 350 °.
In large bowl, combine cereal and peanuts. In small saucepan, heat margarine, peanut butter and cinnamon over low heat until margarine and peanut butter are melted. Stir until blended. Slowly pour over cereal mixture, mixing well. Spread out in a 13x9-inch baking pan. Bake 10-12 minutes, stirring occasionally. Cool.

Nutrition Facts

Serving Size 1/2 cup (55g)
Servings Per Container 8

Amount Per Serving

Calories 270 Calories from Fat 160

	% Daily Value
Total Fat 18g	28%
Saturated Fat 3.5g	18%
Trans Fat 0g	
Cholesterol 0mg	0%
Sodium 85mg	4%
Total Carbohydrate 23g	8%
Dietary Fiber 4g	16%
Sugars 2g	
Protein 9g	

JULI'S SACRED HEART SOUP

Number of Servings: 6

30 oz	No salt added stewed tomatoes	**2 c**	Carrots, chopped
1/3 c	Green onions, tops and bulbs, chopped	**1-1/2 c**	Green bell peppers, chopped
1	15 oz can of fat free reduced sodium beef broth	**1 tsp**	Original blend Mrs. Dash®
		1/2 tsp	Ground black pepper
1 pkg	Chicken noodle soup, dry mix	**1 Tbs**	Fresh parsley, chopped
2 c	Celery, diced	**2 Tbs**	Low sodium Worcestershire sauce
2 c	Green beans	**1 tsp**	Hot pepper sauce

Place vegetables in stock pot; cover with water and boil for 10 minutes. Add tomatoes, soup mix and beef broth. Add spices and stir. Reduce heat to simmer and continue to cook until veggies are tender.

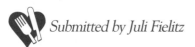 *Submitted by Juli Fielitz*

Nutrition Facts

Serving Size 1 cup (386g)
Servings Per Container 6

Amount Per Serving

Calories 100   Calories from Fat 5

	% Daily Value
Total Fat 0.5g	1%
Saturated Fat 0g	0%
Trans Fat 0g	
Cholesterol 5mg	2%
Sodium 360mg	15%
Total Carbohydrate 20g	7%
Dietary Fiber 6g	24%
Sugars 10g	
Protein 4g	

ASPARAGUS SALAD

Number of Servings: 6

1 lb	Asparagus, trimmed	**1 Tbs**	Sesame seeds, toasted
2 Tbs	Water	**1 tsp**	Fresh ginger root, minced
4 c	Mixed salad greens	**1/4 c**	Slivered almonds, toasted
1/3 c	Balsamic vinegar		
2 Tbs	Orange juice		
2 Tbs	Apricot preserves		
2 Tbs	Pineapple preserves		

Place asparagus and water in a microwave safe 11x7-inch baking dish. Cover and microwave on high for 2-3 minutes or until crisp-tender. Drain and immediately place asparagus in ice water. Drain and pat dry.

Place salad greens on a serving platter; top with asparagus. In a small bowl, mix the vinegar, orange juice, preserves, sesame seeds and minced ginger. Drizzle over salad. Sprinkle with toasted almonds.

Nutrition Facts

Serving Size 1/2 c (155g)
Servings Per Container 6

Amount Per Serving

Calories 100   Calories from Fat 30

	% Daily Value
Total Fat 3.5g	5%
Saturated Fat 0g	0%
Trans Fat 0g	
Cholesterol 0mg	0%
Sodium 20mg	1%
Total Carbohydrate 16g	5%
Dietary Fiber 3g	12%
Sugars 12g	
Protein 4g	

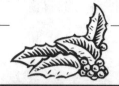

SWEET POTATO SALAD

Number of Servings: 8

2 lb	Sweet potatoes	**1-1/2 c**	Celery, diced
1 c	Fat free mayonnaise	**2/3 c**	Green onions, tops and bulbs, chopped
2 tsp	Dijon mustard		
2	Hard boiled Omega-3 eggs, chopped	**1 tsp**	Ground cinnamon

Place sweet potatoes in a large saucepan and cover with water. Cover and boil gently, about 30-45 minutes, until the potatoes can be easily pierced with the tip of a sharp knife. Drain. When potatoes are cool, peel and dice.

In a large bowl, combine mayonnaise, mustard and salt. Stir in eggs, celery and onions. Sprinkle with cinnamon. Add potatoes; stir gently to mix. Cover and refrigerate for 2-4 hours.

Nutrition Facts

Serving Size 1/2 cup (203g)
Servings Per Container 8

Amount Per Serving

Calories 160   Calories from Fat 25

	% Daily Value
Total Fat 3g	5%
Saturated Fat 0.5g	3%
Trans Fat 0g	
Cholesterol 95mg	32%
Sodium 340mg	14%
Total Carbohydrate 28g	9%
Dietary Fiber 5g	20%
Sugars 7g	
Protein 5g	

CRANBERRY SALAD

Number of Servings: 8

3 c   Fresh cranberries
1   Orange, seedless
1-1/2 c Splenda®
1   Small box of sugar
         free lemon gelatin
1   Small box of sugar
         free cherry gelatin

2 c   Water
1/2 c   Canned pineapple
         tidbits with juice
1 c   Black walnuts,
         chopped

In a food processor, combine the cranberries and the orange (rind and all). Process for 30 seconds. In a medium bowl, combine cranberry/orange mixture and Splenda®. Cover and refrigerate overnight.

In a large bowl, combine the lemon and cherry gelatin with 2 cups boiling water. Chill until just before gelatin starts to set (about 20 minutes). Combine the cranberry/orange mixture, chopped nuts, chopped pineapple and gelatin. Refrigerate at least 4 hours before serving.

Nutrition Facts	
Serving Size 1/4 cup (156g)	
Servings Per Container 8	
Amount Per Serving	
Calories 160 Calories from Fat 80	
	% Daily Value
Total Fat 9g	14%
Saturated Fat 0.5g	3%
Trans Fat 0g	
Cholesterol 0mg	0%
Sodium 20mg	1%
Total Carbohydrate 16g	5%
Dietary Fiber 4g	16%
Sugars 6g	
Protein 4g	

Use 2 egg whites or 1/4 cup egg substitute instead of one whole egg.

CONFETTI SALAD

Number of Servings: 2

1/2 c	Canned black beans, rinsed and drained
1 Tbs	Frozen corn, rinsed and drained
1 Tbs	Avocado, diced
2 Tbs	Yellow bell pepper, diced
2 Tbs	No salt added diced tomato
1 Tbs	Red bell pepper, diced
1 Tbs	Fresh green onion, bulbs only, chopped
1 tsp	Extra virgin olive oil
1/4 tsp	Ground cumin
1/4 tsp	Ground black pepper
1/8 tsp	Salt substitute

Combine all ingredients in a bowl. Serve chilled or at room temperature.

Nutrition Facts

Serving Size 1/2 cup (111g)
Servings Per Container 2

Amount Per Serving

Calories 80   Calories from Fat 30

	% Daily Value
Total Fat 3g	5%
Saturated Fat 0g	0%
Trans Fat 0g	
Cholesterol 0mg	0%
Sodium 150mg	6%
Total Carbohydrate 12g	4%
Dietary Fiber 4g	16%
Sugars 2g	
Protein 3g	

CINNAMON COFFEE CAKE

Number of Servings: 24

1	Box of light yellow cake mix	**1/2 c**	Unsweetened applesauce
1	Small box of sugar free instant vanilla pudding	**1 c**	Water
1	Small box of sugar free instant butterscotch pudding	**1 tsp**	Vanilla extract
		1 c	Splenda® brown sugar blend
1 c	Egg substitute	**1/4 c**	Pecans, chopped
1/4 c	Canola oil	**1 Tbs**	Ground cinnamon

Preheat oven to 375°. In a mixing bowl, combine first 8 ingredients. Beat on low to medium speed for 2 minutes; set aside. In a small bowl, combine Splenda® brown sugar blend, nuts and cinnamon. Pour half of batter into a 9x13-inch baking dish sprayed with cooking spray. Sprinkle half of topping over batter. Pour in the remaining batter and cover with the remaining topping. Bake for 20 minutes. Reduce heat to 325° and bake for 20 minutes. Allow cake to cool 10 minutes before serving.

Nutrition Facts

Serving Size 2-inch square (70g)
Servings Per Container 24

Amount Per Serving	
Calories 260 Calories from Fat 130	
	% Daily Value
Total Fat 15g	23%
Saturated Fat 1.5g	8%
Trans Fat 0g	
Cholesterol 0mg	0%
Sodium 180mg	8%
Total Carbohydrate 20g	7%
Dietary Fiber 1g	4%
Sugars 9g	
Protein 2g	

FRITTATA

Number of Servings: 8

1 c	Egg substitute	**12 oz**	Asparagus, cut into
1	Omega-3 egg		1″ pieces
2 Tbs	Fat free half and half	**2**	Roma tomatoes
1/4 tsp	Ground black pepper	**2 oz**	Fontina cheese
2 tsp	Extra virgin olive oil		
1 Tbs	Trans fat free		
	margarine		

Preheat broiler. Whisk together the eggs, half and half and pepper in a medium bowl.

Slice and seed the tomatoes. Heat oil and margarine in a 9-1/2-inch diameter nonstick ovenproof skillet over medium heat. Add the asparagus and sauté until crisp-tender, about 2 minutes. Raise the heat to medium-high, add the tomatoes and sauté 2 minutes longer.

Nutrition Facts

Serving Size 2-inch wedge (115g)
Servings Per Container 8

Amount Per Serving

Calories 90   Calories from Fat 50

	% Daily Value
Total Fat 5g	8%
Saturated Fat 2g	10%
Trans Fat 0g	
Cholesterol 50mg	17%
Sodium 125mg	5%
Total Carbohydrate 3g	1%
Dietary Fiber 1g	4%
Sugars 2g	
Protein 7g	

Pour the egg mixture over the asparagus mixture and cook for a few minutes until the eggs start to set. Sprinkle the cheese over the mixture and reduce heat to medium-low, cooking until the frittata is almost set but the top is still runny, about 2 minutes.

Place the skillet under the broiler and broil until the top is set and golden brown, about 5 minutes. Remove from broiler and let stand for 2 minutes. Slice and serve either hot or at room temperature.

HEARTY BREAKFAST CASSEROLE

Number of Servings: 12

16	Slices of whole wheat bread, crust removed	**4**	Omega-3 eggs
		4	Egg whites
		1 c	1% milk
8 oz	Low fat low sodium cheddar cheese, shredded	**1 tsp**	Salt substitute
		14 oz	Low fat turkey sausage, crumbled

Preheat oven to 375°. Spray a 9x12-inch baking dish with cooking spray. Place half of bread on bottom, then cover with half of turkey sausage and half of cheese. Repeat layers, ending with cheese. In a small bowl, mix eggs, egg whites, milk and salt substitute. Pour over casserole. Cover casserole and refrigerate overnight. Bake for 45 minutes.

Nutrition Facts

Serving Size 1/2 cup (208g)
Servings Per Container 12

Amount Per Serving	
Calories 250	Calories from Fat 60

	% Daily Value
Total Fat 7g	11%
Saturated Fat 2.5g	13%
Trans Fat 0g	
Cholesterol 90mg	30%
Sodium 570mg	24%
Total Carbohydrate 20g	7%
Dietary Fiber 3g	12%
Sugars 10g	
Protein 26g	

Here are a few benefits of exercise:
- *Increases energy*
- *Burns fat and calories*
- *Improves mood*
- *Protects against heart disease*

HALIBUT WITH CRAB SAUCE

Number of Servings: 4

24 oz	Halibut	**3/4 c**	Fat free reduced sodium chicken broth
1/4 tsp	Salt substitute		
1/4 tsp	Ground black pepper	**1/3 c**	Skim milk
2 tsp	Trans fat free margarine	**1/2 c**	Steamed crab
		2 Tbs	Lemon juice
2 Tbs	Trans fat free margarine	**1/4 tsp**	Dill weed
		1/4 c	Low fat Swiss cheese, shredded
3 Tbs	All purpose flour		

Preheat oven to 350°. Place each fillet in an individual broiler-proof serving dish. Sprinkle with salt substitute and pepper. Melt 2 teaspoons margarine; drizzle over each fillet. Bake, uncovered, for 15-20 minutes or until fish flakes easily.

In a small saucepan coated with nonstick cooking spray, melt remaining margarine. Stir in flour until smooth; add broth and milk. Bring to a boil cooking and stirring for 1-2 minutes or until thickened. Stir in crab, lemon juice and dill. Remove from heat and stir in cheese until melted. Pour over halibut and broil 4-6 inches from heat for 3-4 minutes or until lightly browned.

Nutrition Facts

Serving Size 6 ounce fillet and 1/3 cup sauce (274g)
Servings Per Container 4

Amount Per Serving

Calories 300 Calories from Fat 90

	% Daily Value
Total Fat 11g	17%
Saturated Fat 2.5g	13%
Trans Fat 0g	
Cholesterol 70mg	23%
Sodium 310mg	13%
Total Carbohydrate 6g	2%
Dietary Fiber 0g	0%
Sugars 1g	
Protein 42g	

MIMI'S SHRIMP SCAMPI

Number of Servings: 4

2 lb Large cooked shrimp
1/4 c Extra virgin olive oil
1/4 c Trans fat free margarine
1/4 c Minced garlic

2 tsp Fresh basil leaves, chopped
1/4 c Fresh lemon juice
1/8 tsp Ground black pepper

Heat oil and butter. Add garlic and basil; sauté 1 minute. Add shrimp and cook 3-5 minutes until pink. Stir in lemon juice and pepper. Serve over whole wheat pasta.

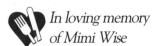 *In loving memory of Mimi Wise*

Nutrition Facts

Serving Size 1/2 cup (231g)
Servings Per Container 4

Amount Per Serving	
Calories 430 Calories from Fat 240	
	% Daily Value
Total Fat 26g	40%
Saturated Fat 5g	25%
Trans Fat 0g	
Cholesterol 335mg	112%
Sodium 480mg	20%
Total Carbohydrate 4g	1%
Dietary Fiber 0g	0%
Sugars 0g	
Protein 36g	

SHRIMP PRIMAVERA

Number of Servings: 12

14 oz	Whole wheat spaghetti	**1 lb**	Medium shrimp, peeled and deveined
1/2 c	Extra virgin olive oil		
3 tsp	Minced garlic	**1 Tbs**	Lemon juice
1/2 tsp	Lemon peel, finely grated	**1/2 tsp**	Salt substitute
		1/8 tsp	Ground black pepper
1	Carrot, cut into 2-inch strips	**2 Tbs**	Fresh basil, chopped
1	Red bell pepper, cut into 2-inch strips	**2 Tbs**	Fresh parsley, chopped

Cook spaghetti according to directions. Meanwhile, heat oil in large skillet, cook and stir garlic and lemon peel about 30 seconds; add vegetables and shrimp. Cook and stir over medium heat until shrimp turn pink, about 3-5 minutes. Sprinkle with lemon juice, salt and pepper. Stir in basil and parsley. Spoon over pasta and toss well.

Nutrition Facts

Serving Size 1/2 cup (177g)
Servings Per Container 12

Amount Per Serving	
Calories 400 Calories from Fat 150	
	% Daily Value
Total Fat 16g	25%
Saturated Fat 2.5g	13%
Trans Fat 0g	
Cholesterol 130mg	43%
Sodium 135mg	6%
Total Carbohydrate 41g	14%
Dietary Fiber 7g	28%
Sugars 3g	
Protein 25g	

Reward yourself. Set weekly exercise goals and reward yourself at the end of the week if you have completed your goals. Rewards could include a nice bubble bath, a new top, a facial or massage.

MEDITERRANEAN ROAST TURKEY

Number of Servings: 8

2 c	White onion, chopped	**1/2 tsp**	Salt substitute
4 oz	Black olives, pitted	**1/4 tsp**	Ground black pepper
1/2 c	Sun dried tomatoes, drained	**4 lbs**	Turkey breast tenderloin
2 Tbs	Lemon juice	**1/2 c**	Fat free reduced sodium chicken broth
1-1/2 tsp	Minced garlic		
1 tsp	Italian seasoning blend	**3 Tbs**	All purpose flour

Combine first 9 ingredients in a crock pot. Add 1/4 cup chicken broth. Cover and cook on LOW for 7 hours.

Combine remaining 1/4 cup broth and flour in a small bowl; stir with a whisk until smooth. Add broth mixture to crock pot. Cover and cook on LOW for 30 minutes.

To serve, cut turkey into slices.

Nutrition Facts

Serving Size 4 ounces turkey and 1/3 cup onion mixture (309g)
Servings Per Container 8

Amount Per Serving

Calories 310   Calories from Fat 60

	% Daily Value
Total Fat 7g	11%
Saturated Fat 0g	0%
Trans Fat 0g	
Cholesterol 90mg	30%
Sodium 300mg	13%
Total Carbohydrate 9g	3%
Dietary Fiber 1g	4%
Sugars 2g	
Protein 57g	

MIKE'S LASAGNA

Number of Servings: 15

2 lb	99% fat free ground turkey breast	**1-1/2 tsp**	Garlic powder
3/4 c	White onion, chopped	**16 oz**	Light mozzarella cheese, shredded
45 oz	Low sodium tomato sauce	**8 oz**	Parmesan, mozzarella and romano cheese, finely shredded
4-1/2 tsp	Italian herb seasoning	**6**	Pieces of whole wheat pasta lasagna noodles
3 tsp	Fresh basil leaves, chopped	**1/2 c**	Fat free ricotta cheese
3 tsp	Anise seeds		
2 tsp	Chili powder		

Preheat oven to 375°. Cook turkey and onions and drain any fat. Combine tomato sauce with spices and simmer 15 minutes; stirring occasionally. Boil lasagna noodles until tender. Drain and rinse. In a 9x13-inch baking dish, layer noodles, meat, onions, sauce, then cheeses. Repeat in same order. Bake 20-25 minutes in oven. It tastes best when served the next day.

Nutrition Facts

Serving Size 3/4 cup (219g)
Servings Per Container 15

Amount Per Serving

Calories 270   Calories from Fat 90

	% Daily Value
Total Fat 10g	15%
Saturated Fat 5g	25%
Trans Fat 0g	
Cholesterol 50mg	17%
Sodium 440mg	18%
Total Carbohydrate 17g	6%
Dietary Fiber 3g	12%
Sugars 1g	
Protein 31g	

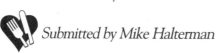

Submitted by Mike Halterman

JAY'S PORK TENDERLOIN SUPPER

Number of Servings: 2

6 oz	Pork tenderloin, sliced into 1-inch medallions	**1/2 c**	Apples, sliced
2 Tbs	Extra virgin olive oil	**1 tsp**	Trans fat free margarine
1/3 c	Brown rice	**1 tsp**	Sugar
2 Tbs	White onion, chopped	**1/4 tsp**	Ground cinnamon
1 c	Water	**1/2 c**	Apples, peeled and sliced
1 pkg	Instant low sodium chicken bouillon granules		

Preheat oven to 350°. In a large skillet, brown pork tenderloin medallions with olive oil. Set medallions aside on a plate. Reserve 1 tablespoon of hot oil.

In the same skillet, cook rice and onion in reserved olive oil until rice is golden, stirring constantly. Stir in water and bouillon granules. Bring to a boil; stir in chopped apple. Put mixture into a 6-inch square baking dish; arrange medallions on top. Bake covered, for 30 minutes. Combine margarine, sugar and cinnamon. Brush sliced apples with mixture; arrange around tenderloins. Bake uncovered, until apples and pork are tender, about 20 minutes.

Nutrition Facts

Serving Size 3 oz medallions (325g)
Servings Per Container 2

Amount Per Serving	
Calories 320 Calories from Fat 170	
	% Daily Value
Total Fat 19g	29%
Saturated Fat 3.5g	18%
Trans Fat 0g	
Cholesterol 55mg	18%
Sodium 65mg	3%
Total Carbohydrate 19g	6%
Dietary Fiber 2g	8%
Sugars 8g	
Protein 19g	

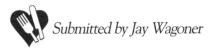 *Submitted by Jay Wagoner*

BUTTERNUT SQUASH AND RED PEPPERS

Number of Servings: 8

7 c	Butternut squash, peeled and cubed	**1 Tbs**	Fresh rosemary
1/2 c	Red sweet bell peppers, chopped	**2 tsp**	Extra virgin olive oil
3 Tbs	Parsley, chopped	**2 tsp**	Minced garlic
		2 Tbs	Parmesan cheese, grated

Preheat oven to 450°. Combine first 6 ingredients; toss well. Place in a 9x13-inch baking dish coated with nonstick cooking spray. Bake for 25-30 minutes or until tender. Sprinkle with cheese before serving.

Nutrition Facts

Serving Size 1 cup (225g)
Servings Per Container 8

Amount Per Serving	
Calories 120	Calories from Fat 15

	% Daily Value
Total Fat 2g	3%
Saturated Fat 0g	0%
Trans Fat 0g	
Cholesterol 0mg	0%
Sodium 30mg	1%
Total Carbohydrate 26g	9%
Dietary Fiber 4g	16%
Sugars 5g	
Protein 3g	

When baking, use fruit purées, applesauce or plain non fat yogurt instead of oil.

BAKED SWEET POTATO CASSEROLE

Number of Servings: 8

5	Sweet potatoes	**2 Tbs**	Trans fat free
1	Omega-3 egg		margarine
3/4 c	Skim milk	**1 Tbs**	Ground cinnamon
2 Tbs	Splenda®		

Preheat oven to 350°. Bake, peel, then mash potatoes; stir in remaining ingredients, mixing until smooth. Pour into 2-quart covered casserole dish sprayed with nonstick cooking spray. Cover and bake approximately one hour. Chopped pecans can be added, if desired.

Nutrition Facts

Serving Size 1/2 cup (116g)
Servings Per Container 8

Amount Per Serving	
Calories 110	Calories from Fat 25

	% Daily Value
Total Fat 3g	5%
Saturated Fat 1g	5%
Trans Fat 0g	
Cholesterol 25mg	8%
Sodium 80mg	3%
Total Carbohydrate 19g	6%
Dietary Fiber 3g	12%
Sugars 5g	
Protein 3g	

BROCCOLI CASSEROLE

Number of Servings: 8

1 pkg	Frozen chopped broccoli, thawed and drained	**8 oz**	2% reduced fat cheddar cheese, shredded
3/4 c	Egg substitute	**1 Tbs**	All purpose flour
12 oz	Fat free cottage cheese	**1/4 tsp**	Salt substitute
		1/2 tsp	Ground black pepper

Preheat oven to 350°. Mix egg substitute, flour, salt substitute and pepper. Add cottage cheese, broccoli and cheddar cheese, reserving some cheese to sprinkle on top. Place in a 2-quart casserole dish sprayed with cooking spray. Cover with remaining cheese. Bake for 1 hour.

Nutrition Facts

Serving Size 1/2 cup (99g)
Servings Per Container 8

Amount Per Serving

Calories 100   Calories from Fat 20

	% Daily Value
Total Fat 2g	3%
Saturated Fat 1.5g	8%
Trans Fat 0g	
Cholesterol 10mg	3%
Sodium 260mg	11%
Total Carbohydrate 4g	1%
Dietary Fiber 0g	0%
Sugars 2g	
Protein 14g	

Don't feel you need to do exercises that you don't enjoy. Pick something that you find fun, such as swimming, rollerblading, skipping, rock climbing or cycling. Everyone is different, so pick something that you enjoy!

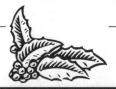

CRANBERRY-ONION RELISH

Number of Servings: 8

1/3 c	White onion, chopped	**2 Tbs**	Splenda®
2 tsp	Minced garlic	**2 Tbs**	Water
2 c	Fresh cranberries	**2 tsp**	Apple cider vinegar
1/4 c	Splenda®		

Spray non-aluminum pan with cooking spray and place on medium heat. Add minced onion and garlic and sauté. Stir in cranberries, 1/4 cup plus 2 tablespoons Splenda® and water. Bring to a low boil and cook 3-5 minutes until cranberries pop and the mixture thickens. Have lid handy to shield mixture but do not close pan. Stir until thickened; then stir in vinegar. Remove from heat. Cool to room temperature. Cover and chill. Relish can be served with meat or chicken.

Nutrition Facts

Serving Size 2 tablespoons (41g)
Servings Per Container 8

Amount Per Serving

Calories 25   Calories from Fat 0

	% Daily Value
Total Fat 0g	0%
Saturated Fat 0g	0%
Trans Fat 0g	
Cholesterol 0mg	0%
Sodium 0mg	0%
Total Carbohydrate 6g	2%
Dietary Fiber 1g	4%
Sugars 3g	
Protein 0g	

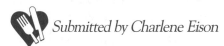 *Submitted by Charlene Eison*

SOURDOUGH STUFFING WITH PEARS AND SAUSAGE

Number of Servings: 12

4	Slices of sourdough bread	**2**	Fresh pears, cubed
4	Slices of whole wheat bread	**1-1/2 Tbs**	Fresh basil, chopped
2	Links light Italian turkey sausage	**2 tsp**	Tarragon
5 c	White onion, chopped	**1 tsp**	Salt substitute
2 c	Celery, diced	**1-1/2 c**	98% fat free 30% reduced sodium chicken broth
1 c	Carrots, diced	**1/2 tsp**	Ground black pepper
8 oz	Mushrooms, sliced		

Preheat oven to 425°. Arrange bread in a single layer on a baking sheet. Bake for 9 minutes or until golden. Break bread slices into cubes. Place in a large bowl.

Remove casing from sausages. Heat a large nonstick skillet over medium-high heat. Coat pan with cooking spray. Add sausage and cook for 8 minutes or until browned, stirring to crumble; drain fat. Add sausage to bread cubes, tossing to combine. Set aside.

Return pan to medium-high heat. Add onion, celery and carrots; sauté 10 minutes or until onion begins to brown. Stir in mushrooms; cook 4 minutes. Stir in pears, basil, tarragon and salt; cook 4 minutes or until pears begins to soften, stirring occasionally.

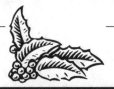

SOURDOUGH STUFFING WITH PEARS AND SAUSAGE

continued

Add pear mixture to bread mixture, tossing gently to combine. Stir in broth and pepper.

Place bread mixture in a 9x13-inch baking dish coated with cooking spray; cover with foil. Bake in oven for 20 minutes. Uncover, bake stuffing an additional 15 minutes or until top of stuffing is crisp.

Nutrition Facts

Serving Size 3/4 cup (220g)
Servings Per Container 12

Amount Per Serving

Calories 170   Calories from Fat 25

	% Daily Value
Total Fat 2.5g	4%
Saturated Fat 0.5g	3%
Trans Fat 0g	
Cholesterol 15mg	5%
Sodium 390mg	16%
Total Carbohydrate 29g	10%
Dietary Fiber 4g	16%
Sugars 9g	
Protein 8g	

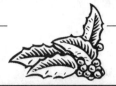

CRANBERRY BEANS

Number of Servings: 8

1 lb	Dried cranberry beans	**1 Tbs**	White pepper
1	Acorn squash	**4**	Bay leaves
2 Tbs	Paprika	**2 tsp**	Ground cumin
1 Tbs	Extra virgin olive oil	**2**	Cans of fat free
3	Yellow onions, diced		reduced sodium
4	Garlic cloves, pressed		chicken broth
			(less 1/2 c)

Rinse beans several times under cold water. Let beans soak 4-12 hours. Pour off water after soaking and rinse again. Add fresh water to cover beans and place in crock pot. Add chicken broth. After 2 hours add bay leaves. Allow to cook on high heat. Meanwhile: Sauté 1/2 cup reserved chicken broth with olive oil, diced onion, garlic and paprika. The mixture should be reddish brown throughout. Add to crock pot with beans. Cut acorn squash in half; place cut side down in a glass dish with 1-inch of water and microwave for 3 minutes on high. Cook until soft and meat is easily removed from skin. Squash is done when it easily mashes with fork. Repeat with other half of

CRANBERRY BEANS

continued

squash. Place squash in a blender to liquefy. Add to crock pot. Add cumin and white pepper. Cook three hours on low heat.

Serve as a soup with liquid, or drained – over brown rice, a whole wheat bread product or whole grain cornbread.

Nutrition Facts	
Serving Size 1/2 cup (249g)	
Servings Per Container 8	
Amount Per Serving	
Calories 160 Calories from Fat 30	
	% Daily Value
Total Fat 3.5g	5%
Saturated Fat 0g	0%
Trans Fat 0g	
Cholesterol 0mg	0%
Sodium 170mg	7%
Total Carbohydrate 28g	9%
Dietary Fiber 9g	36%
Sugars 4g	
Protein 7g	

Acorn-shaped squash is one of the most widely available among the small winter squash. It measures about 6 inches around and weighs 1 to 2 pounds. Acorn squash is a good source of calcium. Baking is an excellent way to bring out the flavor of this squash.

BREAD STUFFING

Number of Servings: 6

15 oz Fat free reduced
sodium chicken broth
1/4 c Celery, diced
1/4 c Red onion, chopped
1/4 c Mushrooms, sliced

6 Slices of whole
grain bread
1/2 tsp Poultry seasoning
1/2 tsp Ground sage
1/2 tsp Ground black pepper

Preheat oven to 325°. Bring chicken broth to a boil. Add celery, onion and mushrooms; simmer for 5 minutes. Cut bread into cubes. Combine the bread cubes and seasonings. Pour broth mixture over bread and toss gently until moistened. Bake in an 8x8-inch dish for 25-30 minutes, until brown on top. (Optional: You can add variety by adding zucchini, peppers, fruits or 1/4 cup nuts.) You may need to prepare additional "moist" ingredients as you add dry ingredients to the recipe.

Nutrition Facts	
Serving Size 3/4 cup (120g)	
Servings Per Container 6	
Amount Per Serving	
Calories 70	Calories from Fat 5
	% Daily Value
Total Fat 0.5g	1%
Saturated Fat 0g	0%
Trans Fat 0g	
Cholesterol 0mg	0%
Sodium 240mg	10%
Total Carbohydrate 15g	5%
Dietary Fiber 5g	20%
Sugars 1g	
Protein 3g	

CRANBERRY WALNUT MUFFINS

Number of Servings: 12

1 c	Whole grain shredded wheat cereal	**1/4 tsp**	Salt substitute
1-1/2 c	1% milk	**1**	Omega 3-egg
1 c	Fresh cranberries	**1/4 c**	Canola oil
1-1/2 c	Whole wheat flour	**1-1/2 Tbs**	Fresh orange peel, grated
1/2 c	Sugar	**3/4 c**	Walnuts, chopped
1 Tbs	Baking powder		

Preheat oven to 400°. Spray muffin tins or line with paper liners. Combine shredded wheat and milk in small mixing bowl and allow to soften for 5 minutes. Pick through cranberries and remove all stems and shriveled berries. If using frozen berries, do not thaw before using. Set aside 1/4 cup of flour to toss with walnuts and cranberries. Combine remaining flour, sugar, baking powder and salt in a large mixing bowl using a fork or whisk. Add egg, oil and orange zest to shredded wheat mixture. Stir to combine. Pour milk/shredded wheat mixture into dry ingredients and stir only until moistened. Mix reserved flour in with walnuts and cranberries, gently fold into batter. Spoon batter into muffin cups. Bake approximately 20 minutes or until center comes out clean. Serve warm.

Nutrition Facts

Serving Size 1 muffin (84g)
Servings Per Container 12

Amount Per Serving

Calories 200 Calories from Fat 100

	% Daily Value
Total Fat 11g	17%
Saturated Fat 1g	5%
Trans Fat 0g	
Cholesterol 20mg	7%
Sodium 125mg	5%
Total Carbohydrate 24g	8%
Dietary Fiber 3g	12%
Sugars 9g	
Protein 5g	

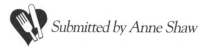 *Submitted by Anne Shaw*

TOASTED ALMOND GRANOLA

Number of Servings: 16

3 c	Old fashioned oats	**1/8 c**	Honey
1/2 c	Toasted wheat germ	**2 tsp**	Canola oil
4 oz	Powdered skim milk	**2 tsp**	Vanilla extract
1/2 c	Slivered almonds	**1/2 tsp**	Almond extract
1/4 c	Brown sugar, packed	**1/4 c**	Golden raisins
2 Tbs	Sunflower kernels	**3 oz**	Dried apricots
1/4 tsp	Salt substitute	**1/3 c**	Dried cranberries
1/3 c	Orange juice		

Preheat oven to 450°. In a large bowl, combine the first 7 ingredients. In a saucepan, combine the orange juice, honey and oil. Heat for 3-4 minutes over medium heat until honey is dissolved. Remove from heat; stir in extracts. Pour over oat mixture; stir to coat.

Place in a 15x10-inch baking pan coated with nonstick cooking spray. Bake for 20-25 minutes or until crisp, stirring every 10 minutes. Remove and cool completely on a wire rack. Stir in fruit. Store in an airtight container. Serve with nonfat plain yogurt if desired.

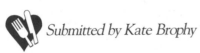 *Submitted by Kate Brophy*

Nutrition Facts

Serving Size 1/2 cup (53g)
Servings Per Container 16

Amount Per Serving

Calories 180   Calories from Fat 40

	% Daily Value
Total Fat 4.5g	7%
Saturated Fat 0g	0%
Trans Fat 0g	
Cholesterol 0mg	0%
Sodium 45mg	2%
Total Carbohydrate 30g	10%
Dietary Fiber 3g	12%
Sugars 13g	
Protein 7g	

CRUSTLESS PUMPKIN PIE

Number of Servings: 8

1	Omega-3 egg, slightly beaten	**1/4 c**	Splenda®
1	16 oz can pumpkin	**1 tsp**	Ground cinnamon
		1/2 tsp	Ground ginger
1/2 c	Sugar	**1/4 tsp**	Ground cloves
		12 oz	Evaporated skim milk

Preheat oven to 425°. Combine ingredients in order listed. Pour into an 8-inch pie plate sprayed with cooking spray. Bake 15 minutes. Reduce oven temperature to 350° and bake an additional 45 minutes or until knife inserted in center of pie comes out clean. Cool. Serve with fat free whipped topping.

Nutrition Facts

Serving Size 1/8 of pie (114g)
Servings Per Container 8

Amount Per Serving

Calories 90   Calories from Fat 5

% Daily Value

Total Fat 1g	2%
Saturated Fat 0g	0%
Trans Fat 0g	
Cholesterol 25mg	8%
Sodium 55mg	2%
Total Carbohydrate 18g	6%
Dietary Fiber 3g	12%
Sugars 14g	
Protein 4g	

MANDARIN ORANGE CREAM CHEESE MUFFINS

Number of Servings: 12

3 Tbs	Trans fat free margarine	**3/4 c**	All purpose flour
1/2 c	Sugar	**1 tsp**	Baking powder
1/3 c	Light cream cheese	**1/2 tsp**	Salt substitute
1/4 c	Egg Substitute	**1/2 c**	1% milk
1	Omega-3 egg	**1 c**	Canned mandarin oranges in light syrup, drained
3/4 c	Whole wheat flour		
1 tsp	Orange flavoring		

Preheat oven to 350°. Coat 12 cup muffin pan with canola cooking spray or line with cupcake liners. Beat margarine and 1/3 cup light cream cheese with an electric mixer on medium speed. Add sugar and beat until creamy. Beat in egg, then egg substitute. Beat in orange flavoring.

Whisk together whole wheat flour, all purpose flour, baking powder and salt substitute. Add half of flour mixture to margarine mixture, then half of the milk. Add in remaining flour mixture, then remaining milk. Gently stir in mandarin oranges.

Fill each muffin cup with 1/3 cup of batter. Bake in center of oven for 15-20 minutes or until cooked through. Cool. Refrigerate in a covered container.

Nutrition Facts

Serving Size 1 muffin (68g)
Servings Per Container 12

Amount Per Serving	
Calories 130 Calories from Fat 35	
	% Daily Value
Total Fat 4g	6%
Saturated Fat 1.5g	8%
Trans Fat 0g	
Cholesterol 20mg	7%
Sodium 100mg	4%
Total Carbohydrate 21g	7%
Dietary Fiber 2g	8%
Sugars 8g	
Protein 4g	

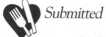 *Submitted by Anne Shaw*

WHOLE WHEAT HOLIDAY COOKIES

Number of Servings: 36

1/2 c	Splenda®	**3 Tbs**	Skim milk
1/2 c	Sugar	**1 Tbs**	Fresh lemon peel
1 tsp	Baking powder	**1 tsp**	Vanilla extract
1/2 tsp	Salt substitute	**1**	Omega-3 egg
1/2 tsp	Baking soda	**2 c**	Whole wheat flour
1/2 tsp	Ground nutmeg	**2 Tbs**	Splenda®
1/2 c	Trans fat free margarine	**1/2 tsp**	Ground cinnamon

Preheat oven to 375°.
Lightly spoon flour into measuring cup; level off. In a large bowl, combine sugar, 1/2 cup Splenda®, baking powder, salt substitute, soda, nutmeg, margarine, milk, lemon peel, vanilla and egg; blend well. Stir in flour. Cover with plastic wrap; chill dough 30 minutes. Roll out dough on lightly floured surface about 1/8-inch thick. Cut with floured cookie cutters. Place on ungreased cookie sheets 2 inches apart. Combine 2 tablespoons Splenda® and cinnamon; sprinkle over cookies. Bake for 8-10 minutes. Let stand 1 minute; cool on wire racks.

Nutrition Facts

Serving Size 1 cookie (16g)
Servings Per Container 36

Amount Per Serving

Calories 50   Calories from Fat 20

	% Daily Value
Total Fat 2.5g	4%
Saturated Fat 0.5g	3%
Trans Fat 0g	
Cholesterol 5mg	2%
Sodium 55mg	2%
Total Carbohydrate 7g	2%
Dietary Fiber 1g	4%
Sugars 2g	
Protein 1g	

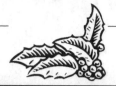

GINGER COOKIES

Number of Servings: 24

1 c	All purpose flour	**1 c**	Sugar
1 c	Whole wheat flour	**1/2 c**	Unsweetened
3/4 c	Crystallized ginger,		applesauce
	chopped	**1/4 c**	Canola oil
1 tsp	Baking powder	**1 tsp**	Lemon rind, grated
1/2 tsp	Baking soda	**1 tsp**	Lemon juice
1/2 tsp	Salt	**1/4 tsp**	Vanilla extract
1/2 tsp	Ground ginger		

Preheat oven to 350°. In a large bowl, combine flours, crystallized ginger, baking powder, baking soda, salt and ground ginger. Stir well with a whisk. Make a well in center of mixture. In a small bowl, combine 3/4 cup sugar, applesauce, canola oil, grated lemon rind, lemon juice and vanilla extract. Add to flour mixture, stirring just until moist; cover and chill dough at least 1 hour.

Nutrition Facts

Serving Size 1 cookie (39g)
Servings Per Container 24

Amount Per Serving

Calories 130   Calories from Fat 20

	% Daily Value
Total Fat 2.5g	4%
Saturated Fat 0g	0%
Trans Fat 0g	
Cholesterol 0mg	0%
Sodium 95mg	4%
Total Carbohydrate 26g	9%
Dietary Fiber 1g	4%
Sugars 14g	
Protein 1g	

Lightly coat hands with flour. Shape dough into 24 balls (2 tablespoons each; dough will be sticky). Roll balls in 1/4 cup sugar. Place on cookie sheet 2 inches apart. Bake for 15 minutes.

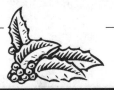

CHERYL'S PUMPKIN CRUNCH

Number of Servings: 12

2	Cans of solid pumpkin	**1-1/2 tsp**	Ground cinnamon
1	Can of evaporated skim milk	**1/2 box**	Dry yellow cake mix
1 c	Splenda®	**3/4 c**	Unsalted light butter
3	Omega-3 eggs	**1-1/2 c**	Walnuts, chopped

Preheat oven to 350°.
Mix together the solid pumpkin, milk, Splenda®, eggs and ground cinnamon. Pour into ungreased 9x13-inch pan. Sprinkle 1/2 box of dry yellow cake mix on top. Pour melted light butter on top of cake mix and spread until evenly distributed; top with walnuts. Bake for 50-60 minutes or until toothpick comes out clean. Let set for 30 minutes.

Nutrition Facts

Serving Size 3/4 cup (158g)
Servings Per Container 12

Amount Per Serving	
Calories 310 Calories from Fat 170	
	% Daily Value
Total Fat 19g	29%
Saturated Fat 5g	25%
Trans Fat 0g	
Cholesterol 65mg	22%
Sodium 170mg	7%
Total Carbohydrate 28g	9%
Dietary Fiber 4g	16%
Sugars 15g	
Protein 10g	

 Submitted by Cheryl Kuhta-Sutter

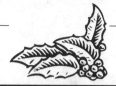

CHOCOLATE RASPBERRY MOUSSE

Number of Servings: 16

2c	Skim milk
1	Small box of sugar free instant chocolate pudding
1 c	Fat free sour cream
1/2 c	Fat free whipped topping
48 oz	Frozen raspberries
16 sq	Low fat graham crackers

In a large bowl, using a whisk, beat pudding mix and milk together until smooth and creamy. Add the sour cream and whipped topping. Whisk until smooth. Fold in 2 cups of raspberries. Pour into a 9x13-inch baking dish; spread evenly with a spatula. Press graham cracker pieces into mousse; distribute evenly. Sprinkle the remaining raspberries over the top. Cover and refrigerate at least 3 hours.

Nutrition Facts

Serving Size 1/3 cup (142g)
Servings Per Container 16

Amount Per Serving	
Calories 90	Calories from Fat 5

	% Daily Value
Total Fat 0.5g	1%
Saturated Fat 0g	0%
Trans Fat 0g	
Cholesterol 0mg	0%
Sodium 80mg	3%
Total Carbohydrate 19g	6%
Dietary Fiber 1g	4%
Sugars 9g	
Protein 3g	

Replace the meat in your chili or other casseroles with extra beans, tofu or tempeh. Experiment with different varieties of beans.

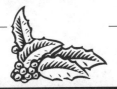

CHOCOLATE CAKE

Number of Servings: 12

5	Egg whites	**1/4 tsp**	Salt substitute
3/4 c	Fat free plain yogurt	**1/2 c**	Splenda®
3 c	Zucchini, grated	**2 tsp**	Ground cinnamon
1/2 c	Unsweetened applesauce	**1/2 tsp**	Cream of tartar
1/2 c	Unsweetened cocoa powder	**1/3 c**	Sugar
		12 oz	Fat free whipped topping
2-1/2 c	Cake flour	**1/4 tsp**	Vanilla extract
1 tsp	Baking soda	**1 Tbs**	Unsweetened cocoa powder
2 tsp	Baking powder		

Preheat oven to 350°. Coat bottom of a 9x13-inch cake pan with cooking spray. Combine all ingredients in large bowl; beat on low speed for 2 minutes, scraping sides of bowl often. Pour mixture into cake pan. Bake for 45-50 minutes or until toothpick inserted into center comes out clean. Cool. Top with fat free whipped topping mixed with a few drops of vanilla. Dust with cocoa powder.

Nutrition Facts

Serving Size 2-inch piece (105g)
Servings Per Container 12

Amount Per Serving

Calories 190   Calories from Fat 5

	% Daily Value
Total Fat 0.5g	1%
Saturated Fat 0g	0%
Trans Fat 0g	
Cholesterol 0mg	0%
Sodium 220mg	9%
Total Carbohydrate 39g	13%
Dietary Fiber 1g	4%
Sugars 11g	
Protein 5g	

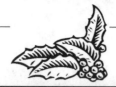

PUNCH BOWL CAKE
Number of Servings: 12

16 oz Fat free whipped topping
1/2 c Fat free sweetened condensed milk
8 oz Low fat cream cheese

2 c Strawberries, sliced
1 c Blueberries
1 Sugar free angel food cake

Mix cool whip, sweetened condensed milk and cream cheese in large bowl; set aside. Wash fruit; set aside. Break up cake into pieces; set aside. Place a single layer of fruit in punch bowl. Next, place a layer of cake, then cover cake with some of the whipped topping mixture. Continue repeating layers ending with fruit.

Nutrition Facts

Serving Size 1/2 cup (129g)
Servings Per Container 12

Amount Per Serving	
Calories 200	Calories from Fat 30

	% Daily Value
Total Fat 3.5g	5%
Saturated Fat 2g	10%
Trans Fat 0g	
Cholesterol 10mg	3%
Sodium 170mg	7%
Total Carbohydrate 33g	11%
Dietary Fiber 1g	4%
Sugars 7g	
Protein 5g	

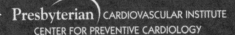

Presbyterian CARDIOVASCULAR INSTITUTE
CENTER FOR PREVENTIVE CARDIOLOGY

MENU PLANS

SEASONS *of the* HEART

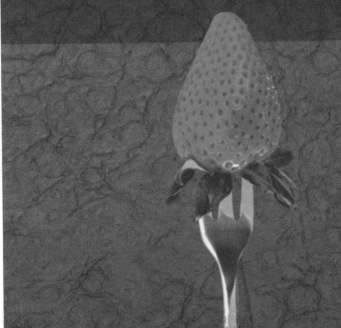

1400 CALORIE MEAL PLAN
Day 1

Breakfast

2	Slices whole wheat toast
1 tsp	Trans fat free margarine
1 Tbs	Sugar free jelly
1/2 c	1% cottage cheese
1/2 c	Canned peaches in own juice
8 oz	Skim milk

Lunch

1/2-6 inch	Whole wheat pita
2 oz	Cooked chicken mixed with
1 Tbs	Light mayonnaise
1	Scallion
1 Tbs	Diced celery
1/2	Sliced zucchini
2 Tbs	Fat free Italian salad dressing to dip zucchini
1 1/4 c	Cubed cantaloupe
	Water or non-caloric beverage

Dinner

4 oz	Cubed salmon
1/2 c	Sliced onion
1 tsp	Olive oil to sauté onion and salmon
1/3 c	No salt added tomato sauce; diluted with 1/3 c water and add during the last few minutes of cooking
10	Small green olives
1 c	Cooked whole wheat pasta
1 c	Cauliflower
	Water or non-caloric beverage

Evening Snack

1 c	Fat free yogurt (sugars less than 11 grams)
1/2 c	Diced fruit packed in own juice

1400 CALORIE MEAL PLAN
Day 2

Breakfast
1	Ziploc Omelet (pg 81)
2	Slices whole wheat bread
1/2 Tbs	Trans fat free margarine
1	Orange
8 oz	Skim milk

Lunch
2	Slices light whole wheat bread
2 oz	Turkey breast
1 oz	Low fat cheese
1 tsp	Light mayonnaise
1	Apple
	Water or non-caloric beverage

Dinner
2	Beef Enchiladas (pg 97)
1/3 c	Black beans
	Water or non-caloric beverage

Evening Snack
2	Low fat graham cracker squares
1 Tbs	Natural peanut butter

1400 CALORIE MEAL PLAN

Day 3

Breakfast

1	Oatmeal Pancake (pg 36)
1 tsp	Trans fat free margarine
1 Tbs	Chopped pecans
2 tsp	Sugar free pancake syrup
1/2 c	Blueberries
8 oz	Skim milk

Lunch

1	Whole tomato, inside scooped out
1/2 c	Tuna Salad (pg 85)
1	Green pepper, sliced in spears
2 Tbs	Fat free ranch dressing to dip spears
8 oz	Skim milk

Dinner

1 1/2 c	Kathy's Chicken Squash Pasta Medley (pg 126)
1 c	Steamed spinach
	Iced tea (sweetened with Splenda®)

Evening Snack

1/4 c	1% cottage cheese
1 c	Strawberries

1600 CALORIE MEAL PLAN

Day 1

Breakfast

2	Slices whole wheat toast
4 tsp	Natural peanut butter
1/2	Small banana
8 oz	Skim milk

Lunch

2	Slices whole wheat bread
2 Tbs	Pimento Cheese Spread (pg 115)
1/2 c	Baby carrots
2 Tbs	Fat free dressing for dipping carrots
	Water or non-caloric beverage

Dinner

1	Cod Picatta Florentine Fillet (pg 84)
2/3 c	Brown rice
1/2 c	Steamed broccoli
	Iced tea (sweetened with Splenda®)

Evening Snack

1/4 c	Cantaloupe
1/4 c	1% cottage cheese

1600 CALORIE MEAL PLAN

Day 2

Breakfast

1 1/2 c	Whole wheat cereal
1	Apple
4 tsp	Natural peanut butter to spread on apple
8 oz	Skim milk

Lunch

1 c	Chicken Strawberry Spinach Salad (pg 79)
	Water or non-caloric beverage

Dinner

	Laura's Chicken in Wine (pg 50)
1 c	Steamed spinach
2/3 c	Brown rice
	Iced tea (sweetened with Splenda®)

Evening Snack

8	Animal crackers
8 oz	Skim milk

1600 CALORIE MEAL PLAN
Day 3

Breakfast

2/3 c	Oatmeal with Apples and Walnuts (pg 80)
1/2 c	Sliced pears
8 oz	Skim milk

Lunch

3 oz	Grilled chicken
1 1/4 c	Wilted Spinach Salad (pg 33)
	Iced tea (sweetened with Splenda®)

Dinner

	Halibut with Crab Sauce (pg 200)
2 c	Garden salad
2 Tbs	Fat free salad dressing
1	Whole wheat dinner roll
	Water or non-caloric beverage

Evening Snack

1 c	Fat free yogurt (sugar less than 11 grams)
1	Peach

1800 CALORIE MEAL PLAN

Day 1

Breakfast

2	Slices whole wheat toast
1	Tomato sliced
1	Omega-3 egg and 3 egg whites (scrambled)
1	Peach
8 oz	Skim milk

Lunch

1 c	Slow Cooked Black Bean Chili (pg 31)
1 c	Garden salad
2 Tbs	Fat free dressing
	Water or non-caloric beverage

Dinner

3/4 c	Mike's Lasagna (pg 204)
1/2 c	Green beans
1	Whole wheat dinner roll
1 tsp	Trans fat free margarine

Evening Snack

2	Chocolate Oatmeal Boiled Cookies (pg 181)
8 oz	Skim milk

1800 CALORIE MEAL PLAN

Day 2

Breakfast

3-4 inch	Hearty Oatmeal Pancakes (pg 151)
1/2 c	Blueberries
2 Tbs	Sugar free pancake syrup
1 c	Decaf coffee or tea

Lunch

1 c	Chicken Broccoli Chowder (pg 147)
1 c	Spinach Salad (pg 150)
	Water or non-caloric beverage

Dinner

1	Orange-Basil Salmon with Green Beans (pg 153)
2/3 c	Whole wheat pasta
1 tsp	Trans fat free margarine
1	Whole wheat dinner roll
8 oz	Skim milk

Evening Snack

1/2 c	Fat free, sugar free pudding
2 Tbs	Fat free whipped topping
1 Tbs	Chopped nuts
8 oz	Skim milk

1800 CALORIE MEAL PLAN
Day 3

Breakfast
1 c	Whole wheat cereal
1/2 c	Berries
1 Tbs	Nuts
8 oz	Skim milk

Lunch
2	Slices whole wheat bread
3 oz	Sliced turkey breast
	Lettuce and tomato
2 tsp	Light mayonnaise
1/2 c	Baby carrots
12	Grapes

Dinner
3 oz	Grilled boneless, skinless chicken breast
1 Tbs	(15 calorie) Barbeque sauce
2/3 c	Brown rice
1 c	Asparagus
1 c	Garden salad
2 Tbs	Fat free salad dressing
1	Kiwi
	Water or non-caloric beverage

Evening Snack
1 c	Fat free yogurt (sugars less than 11 grams)
1/4 c	Berries
1 Tbs	Walnuts

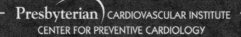

INDEX

SEASONS *of the* HEART

Index

Fish

Poultry

Grains

Brown Rice with Lemon & Shallots	Spring	100
Corn Muffins	Autumn	177
Cranberry Walnut Muffins	Holiday	215
Harvest Muffins	Autumn	175
Muffins	Winter	67
Savory Add-A-Crunch	Autumn	176
Tassajara Granola	Autumn	178
Toasted Almond Granola	Holiday	216
Whole Wheat Carrot Muffins	Summer	134
Wholegrain Muffins	Summer	101
Wild Rice Pilaf	Autumn	174

Desserts

Apple-Peanut Butter Crisp	Autumn	179
Banana Crunch Cake	Winter	71
Blackberry Peach Crisp	Summer	137
Blueberry Gelatin Salad	Summer	135
Brownies	Winter	73
Cappuccino Pudding Cake	Winter	72
Cherry Chocolate Cake	Summer	141
Cheryl's Pumpkin Crunch	Holiday	221
Chocolate Cake	Holiday	223
Chocolate Éclair Cake	Winter	70
Chocolate Oatmeal Boiled Cookies	Autumn	181
Chocolate Pudding Pie	Spring	107
Chocolate Raspberry Mousse	Holiday	222
Cinnamon Add-A-Crunch	Autumn	183
Crustless Pumpkin Pie	Holiday	217
Ginger Cookies	Holiday	220
Easy Jello Dessert	Spring	103
Jordan's Berry Banana Smoothie	Summer	138
Key Lime-Coconut Mini Cheesecakes	Summer	143
Key Lime Pie	Summer	142
Layered Fruit Sensation	Winter	68
Mandarin Orange Cream Cheese Muffins	Holiday	218
Marcia's Marbled Chocolate Banana Bread	Autumn	182
Meme's Squash Pie	Summer	144
Mixed Berry Smoothie	Spring	102
Oatmeal Raisin Cookies	Winter	69
Orange Nut Whole Wheat Cake	Autumn	180
Peach Crisp	Summer	136
Pineapple & Cheese Casserole	Spring	105
Pineapple Angel Lush	Spring	106
Punch Bowl Cake	Holiday	224
Strawberry Angel Food Delight	Summer	140
Strawberry Fruit Pie	Spring	104
Strawberry Pie	Summer	139
Whole Wheat Holiday Cookies	Holiday	219

How to order extra cookbooks

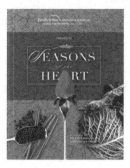

You may order additional copies of this cookbook for $24.00 each ($20.00 cookbook plus $2.50 postage/handling and $1.50 sales tax per book ordered).

Mail your order to:
Presbyterian Center for Preventive Cardiology
125 Baldwin Avenue, Suite 200
Charlotte, NC 28204

Please ship cookbooks to:
Name _____
Address _____
City, State, Zip _____

You can also order by phone at 704-384-5043 using your credit card. For more information, visit our website at www.presbyterian.org.

Enjoy "Seasons of the Heart"? You can also purchase our first cookbook, "Eat Your Heart Out". Call, visit our web site, or use the order form on the next page.

Order copies of our first cookbook, "Eat Your Heart Out"

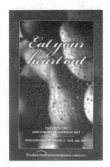

Copies are $24.00 each ($20.00 cookbook plus $2.50 postage/handling and $1.50 sales tax per book ordered).

Mail your order to:
Presbyterian Center for Preventive Cardiology
125 Baldwin Avenue, Suite 200
Charlotte, NC 28204

Please ship cookbooks to:
Name _____
Address _____
City, State, Zip _____

You can also order by phone at 704-384-5043 using your credit card. For more information, visit our website at www.presbyterian.org.

NOTES

NOTES

NOTES